ePractice Kit for

MEDICAL FRONT OFFICE SKILLS

with MedTrak Systems

ELSEVIER
SAUNDERS

ePractice Kit for

MEDICAL FRONT OFFICE SKILLS

with MedTrak Systems

Carol J. Buck, MS, CPC, CPC-H, CCS-P
Program Director, Retired
Medical Secretary Programs
Northwest Technical College
East Grand Forks, Minnesota

Technical Collaborator
Jacqueline Klitz Grass, MA, CPC
Coding Specialist
Grand Forks, North Dakota

Competency Developer
Lyn O'Neal, RMA
Department Chair
Allied Health Department
Skagit Valley College
Mount Vernon, Washington

ELSEVIER
SAUNDERS

3251 Riverport Lane
Maryland Heights, Missouri 63043

ePractice Kit for Medical Front Office Skills with MedTrak Systems   ISBN: 978-1-4377-2722-7
Copyright © 2012 by Saunders, an imprint of Elsevier Inc.

Notices

Knowledge and best practice in this field are constantly changing. As new research and experience broaden our understanding, changes in research methods, professional practices, or medical treatment may become necessary.

Practitioners and researchers must always rely on their own experience and knowledge in evaluating and using any information, methods, compounds, or experiments described herein. In using such information or methods they should be mindful of their own safety and the safety of others, including parties for whom they have a professional responsibility.

With respect to any drug or pharmaceutical products identified, readers are advised to check the most current information provided (i) on procedures featured or (ii) by the manufacturer of each product to be administered, to verify the recommended dose or formula, the method and duration of administration, and contraindications. It is the responsibility of practitioners, relying on their own experience and knowledge of their patients, to make diagnoses, to determine dosages and the best treatment for each individual patient, and to take all appropriate safety precautions.

To the fullest extent of the law, neither the Publisher nor the authors, contributors, or editors, assume any liability for any injury and/or damage to persons or property as a matter of products liability, negligence or otherwise, or from any use or operation of any methods, products, instructions, or ideas contained in the material herein.

ISBN: 978-1-4377-2722-7

Developmental Editor: Diane Chatman
Publishing Services Manager: Pat Joiner-Myers
Cover Designer: Ashley Eberts

Printed in the United States of America

Last digit is the print number: 9   8   7   6   5   4   3   2   1

*This text is dedicated to instructors who give endlessly to others and
make a profound difference in the lives of so many.
Thank you for what you do.*

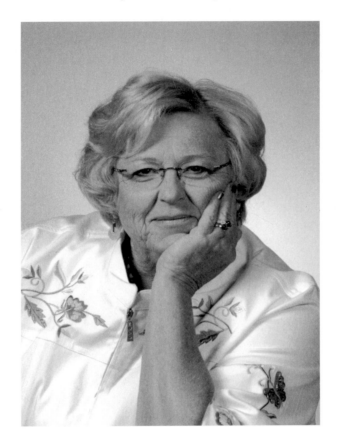

Carol J. Buck

Reviewers

Heidi Aguilar
Medical Transcriptionist
Grand Forks, North Dakota

Donna Maher, MS, CMRS, RHIA
Medical Administrative Program
Renton Technical College
Renton, Washington

Andrea Navajar
Service Specialist
Northwestern Mutual Company
Milwaukee, Wisconsin

Helen Spain, Coordinator
Medical Office Administration
Instructor Office Administration
Wake Technical Community College
Raleigh, North Carolina

Beverly Wheeler, MBA, RHIA, ACS-EM
Consultant, Coding, Auditing & Physician In-Service
Schertz, Texas

Preface

The hub of the modern medical office is the computer. Practice management is accomplished by means of computer software designed to process and store medical records, appointments, billing, and numerous other medical office tasks. Many health care facilities are now paperless, and others are in varying stages of transition to become paperless. There are, however, facilities that remain papered offices. The extent to which you will utilize a computer to accomplish your daily tasks will be determined by the facility in which you are employed, but regardless of the extent of the use of the computer, you will need to be familiar with a wide range of tasks that are standard in the medical office. For example, medical dictation may be transcribed and stored in electronic medium or printed on paper to be filed into the medical record. Either way, you need to be able to transcribe medical dictation, no matter what the terminal storage. The learning is what is important in the process.

As you complete the tasks in this ePractice Kit, you will learn how to accomplish the basic medical office tasks and better prepare yourself to begin your new career in a medical setting.

Success is the sum of small efforts, repeated day in and day out.
—Robert Collier

Contents

Day 7

Day 8

Day 9

Day 10

Appendices

Learning Objectives

Upon completion of this ePractice Kit, you should be able to:

1. Demonstrate basic knowledge of confidentiality and HIPAA regulations.
2. Prepare the appointment schedule for appointment scheduling.
3. Schedule patient appointments according to office rules based on patient need, facility availability, and physician preference.
4. Schedule inpatient and outpatient admissions and procedures.
5. Prepare a daily patient list.
6. Store electronic medical records.
7. Complete a daily bank deposit ticket.
8. Reconcile a bank statement.
9. Post daily entries.
10. Perform accounts receivable procedures.
11. Perform accounts payable procedures.
12. Prepare monthly patient bills.
13. Perform collection procedures.
14. Establish a petty cash fund.
15. Post adjustments.
16. Process a credit balance.
17. Process refunds.
18. Post nonsufficient fund checks.
19. Post collection agency payments.
20. Obtain preauthorization for procedures.
21. Obtain managed care referrals and precertifications.
22. Apply the correct procedural and diagnosis codes for services provided.
23. Prepare insurance claim forms for Medicare, Medicaid, managed care carriers, and private health insurance carriers.
24. Correctly calculate payment for services.
25. Record a variety of telephone messages left on an answering machine.
26. Set up and maintain electronic patient records.
27. Prepare draft documents for your supervisor's review.
28. Demonstrate an understanding of risk management procedures.
29. Perform inventory of equipment.
30. Perform routine maintenance of administrative equipment.
31. Key documents from your supervisor's drafts.
32. Transcribe from several people dictation consisting of medical documents and general correspondence.
33. Maintain an electronic records system.
34. Demonstrate an understanding of the EHR.
35. Exhibit the ability to obtain information from the EHR.

EVOLVE WEBSITE

http://evolve.elsevier.com/Buck/epracticekit/

The Evolve website contains a patient directory, audio files, patient records, and interactive forms required for completion of some tasks. The information on the website is divided by day and subdivided by tasks, such as Day 1, Task 1.3 or Day 6, Task 6.1. To locate records, audio, or forms needed to complete a task, click the link provided for the day the task occurs on, then click the task you are completing.

- **Access to MedTrak Systems**
  Link directly to the virtual South Padre Medical Center/MedTrak Systems software used throughout this book.
- **Audio File**
  MP3 file contains medical dictation information for transcription and telephone messages.
- **Forms Library**
  All the forms used in the internship are available as interactive PDFs for the full experience of working in a paperless medical office.
- **Digital Patient Records**
  Hospital reports to be uploaded into the electronic health record are located on the Evolve site for real-world practice.
- **Patient Directory**
  As a helpful resource, a comprehensive list of patients included in this kit is provided.
- **Quizzes**
  Ten electronic quizzes test your knowledge and can be submitted directly to your instructor.

A WELCOME FROM OUR STAFF

Welcome to the South Padre Medical Center. You will find the Center to be a busy, friendly place to work where your skills, knowledge, and abilities will be appreciated and utilized.

The employees of the Center are here to help you put your education and training into action by performing the tasks that you learned in your educational program. We have been involved in the internship process for more than a decade and see the internship experience as a vital part of your education. We want to help you be successful. You can expect that all employees will treat you as a professional member of the health care team. Mutual respect is absolutely necessary to ensure South Padre Medical Center has an environment conducive to superior patient care. On behalf of each member of the team, we are glad you are here and hope you find your experience with us rewarding.

Your Internship Duties

Your education has prepared you for this internship. Your internship will require you to do a variety of front office tasks in the areas of written correspondence, records management, telephone messages, patient appointments, mail, transcription, insurance claim, travel schedules, banking services, bookkeeping, payroll, and arranging for meetings. Jennifer White, RN, is the office manager and has assigned Gladys Johnson, Medical Office Assistant, to provide your orientation, training, and supervision. You will also spend some time working with Kerri Marshall, CPC, who is the insurance specialist for the Center; however, Gladys Johnson will remain your supervisor throughout the duration of your internship.

Calendar and Work Hours

Your internship covers a two-week period from April 9 to April 20, 2012.

April 2012

Sun	Mon	Tue	Wed	Thur	Fri	Sat
1	2	3	4	5	6	7
8	9	10	11	12	13	14
15	16	17	18	19	20	21
22	23	24	25	26	27	28
29	30					

Your work hours are from 7:45 a.m. to 4:45 p.m. each day. Gladys and you should arrive 15 minutes prior to the start of office hours to open the office and begin answering the telephones promptly at 8 a.m. Kerri Marshall arrives at 8:15 a.m. and works until 5:15 p.m. and covers the reception desk from 4:45 p.m. until 5:15 p.m. The nursing personnel cover the reception desk from 5:15 p.m. until closing.

All staff take an hour lunch break, except on Wednesdays, when everyone takes a half-hour lunch break while three of the physicians are seeing office patients. All staff take a 15-minute break in the morning and afternoon at various times to ensure continuous coverage of all Center services. You will take your breaks at the same time as Gladys takes her breaks. Kerri Marshall covers the reception area for Gladys and you when both of you are on breaks.

Pre-Tasks

Orientation

Note: Supplementary materials for all the activities are located in the Task folders on the companion Evolve site at http://evolve.elsevier.com/Buck/epracticekit/. These folders are labeled first for the Day (such as Day 1, Day 2, etc.), then within each folder, by the Task (such as Task 1.1, Task 1.2, etc.). For example, within the Task folder, in subfolder Day 1, the document labeled Task 1.1 is the Equipment Maintenance and Desk Security Form.

PRE-TASK **1.1**

RISK MANAGEMENT

Supplies Located on Evolve

- Confidentiality Statement

Today, before you begin your internship, Gladys Johnson, the Medical Office Assistant, tells you that she would like to share a very important part of her job with you—risk management. She explains that risk management procedures are used in the Center and are the responsibility of all staff members. *Risk* is defined as any occurrence that may result in injury to a patient, staff member, or visitor or as any liability that could result in financial loss to the Center. A major risk factor to any health care facility is management of patient information, and this is an important aspect of every health care facility member's job. Gladys has been designated the Privacy Officer for the Center and as such is responsible for ensuring that policies and procedures are in place and that all staff members are trained in patient rights and the Health Insurance Portability and Accountability Act of 1996 (HIPAA). The primary function of HIPAA is to provide continuous insurance coverage for employees and their dependents when they change or lose their jobs. Another function of HIPAA is to reduce the costs of managing the exchange of patient data. One part of the management of patient data is standardization of electronic transactions, and the other part is the implementation of security and privacy procedures that ensure confidentiality of patient information. Further, the Act ensures that patients have the legal right to restrict access to their health records and to know who accesses those records. All staff members are responsible for complying with HIPAA and safeguarding all patient information.

Every employee is required to read and sign a confidentiality statement, Figure P-1. Please take a moment to read and sign the statement below.

South Padre Medical Center
Confidentiality Agreement

I understand that all information regarding patients and their health care is considered confidential. Information may be written, verbal or in computerized format. Any information regarding patients that is acquired during the course employed at South Padre Medical Center shall be considered confidential.

I understand that confidential information must never be disclosed for non-employment related purposes. Disclosure of confidential information outside of my assigned duties will constitute unauthorized release of confidential information and can be considered reason for termination of employment.

By signing this document, I acknowledge that I understand this statement and agree to abide by all policies and procedures pertaining to confidentiality of patient information.

_____   _____
Employee signature   Date

_____   _____
Witness Signature   Date

Figure P-1: South Padre Medical Center Confidentiality Agreement (Modified from Potter BP: *Medical office administration: a worktext*, St. Louis, 2010, Saunders.)

Confidentiality is a critically important aspect of your position. The patients' names, addresses, telephone numbers, disorders, and financial information are all examples of confidential information. Even the fact that the patient is a Center patient is confidential. You will be allowed access to patient information on a need-to-know basis. You are not allowed to access patient information that you do not have a reason to access. Do not discuss patient information unless you need to do so to complete your assigned tasks. If you should need to discuss patient information, please do so quietly, being cautious that other patients or staff do not overhear your discussion.

When you receive a request for release of information, you are to verify that the release documentation has the signature of the patient, or in the case of a minor or incompetent patient, the signature of the legal guardian. As an intern or a new employee, you are to ask your supervisor/trainer to verify that the release documentation is correct before releasing any information.

All documentation containing patient information, of any kind, is to be kept from public view. This includes, but is not limited to, appointment schedules, patient records, laboratory/pathology reports, surgery reports, insurance forms, financial information, and telephone logs.

The respect that you show for our patients by keeping their information confidential should also be extended to our physicians. You are a reflection of the Center in all you do and say, especially in what you say about the Center and its staff. Professionalism and respect for the privacy of the physicians and employees of the South Padre Medical Center is an expectation of all Center employees.

Another important component of risk management reduction in the health care setting is for each employee to report any situation that may place patients, employees, or the facility at risk. For example, if you witness any behavior that would be considered risky, such as the odor of alcohol on a fellow employee, you should immediately report the behavior to your supervisor. Also, it is essential that you pay attention to details that may present a risk in the Center, such as a rug with a turned-up corner or a chair that is placed too far into a traffic path in the waiting room. You must be alert to every possible detail in the office to ensure that the office space is as safe as you can make it. Each member of the health care team must assume responsibility for safety in the Center.

PRE-TASK 1.2

ROUTINE MAINTENANCE

 Supplies Located on Evolve

- Equipment Maintenance and Desk Security Form

You are expected to perform routine maintenance on the administrative equipment you use while an intern at the Center. Maintenance supplies are located in the lower right drawer of your desk. At the end of each day, you are to wipe the computer screen with a dry, soft cloth. Never use any type of cleaner on the computer screen because it will damage the screen surface. Use a soft brush to sweep the keyboard at the end of each day. Organize your work and place all papers in the desk drawer at the end of the day, during your breaks, or at any time you leave your desk area. Gladys, Medical Office Assistant, will be your supervisor and will provide you with a key to lock your desk if you need to leave it unattended. Always keep your area clear of patient information that could be seen by others. Clean the top of your desk at the end of each day with spray cleaner.

At the Center, we understand that each intern's knowledge differs when it comes to the operation of the various office equipment. Gladys will provide a demonstration on the operation of all equipment you will be using during your internship. Should the equipment malfunction while you are using it, please contact Gladys.

It's time for you to get started, so first create a folder labeled "Completed Work" (on your computer desktop or jump drive) in which you will save your electronic documents. This folder will serve as the central location for electronic copies of the tasks that you will be performing during your internship. Within your main Completed Work folder, create 10 folders labeled for each of the 10 days of your internship (Day 1, Day 2, Day 3, etc.). Within each Day folder, you will create Task folders. For example, Day 1 has three tasks (Tasks 1.1, 1.2, and 1.3). It makes it much easier to locate your downloaded or saved documents if you make these subfolders. Locate the form labeled "Equipment Maintenance and Desk Security" (Figure P-2) in the Task folder for Day 1, Task 1.1 on the companion Evolve site. Save this form in your newly created Completed Work folder, Day 1, Task 1.1 subfolder. Open the form and key in your name on the line provided. At the end of each day of your internship, check off that you have performed all necessary maintenance of your equipment and that you have secured your desk. At the end of your internship, you will print this form and turn it in to Gladys as verification that you have adhered to the Center's policy regarding equipment maintenance and desk security.

Equipment Maintenance and Desk Security

INTERN: _____

INTERNSHIP DATES:____April 9 - April 20, 2012_____

SUPERVISOR:_____Gladys Johnson_____

DATE	MAINTAINED EQUIPMENT	SECURED DESK
April 09		
April 10		
April 11		
April 12		
April 13		
April 16		
April 17		
April 18		
April 19		
April 20		

Figure P-2: Equipment Maintenance and Desk Security form

PRE-TASK **1.3**

INTRODUCTION TO SOUTH PADRE MEDICAL CENTER

You are now ready to begin your two-week internship at the South Padre Medical Center, a medical office located in South Padre, Texas. The Center is a partnership of four physicians affiliated with Texas Health Corporation, a managed care corporation located in Houston, Texas. Figure P-3 displays the organizational structure of the Center and the affiliation with Texas Health Corporation.

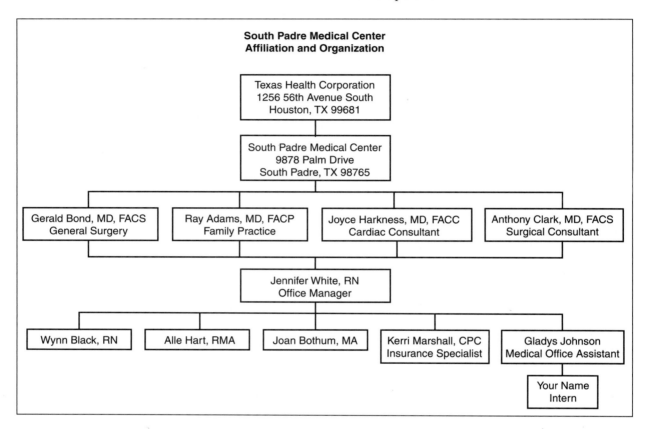

Figure P-3: Organizational structure of the South Padre Medical Center

South Padre Medical Center, shown in Figure P-4, is located at 9878 Palm Drive in South Padre in the South Padre Medical Complex.

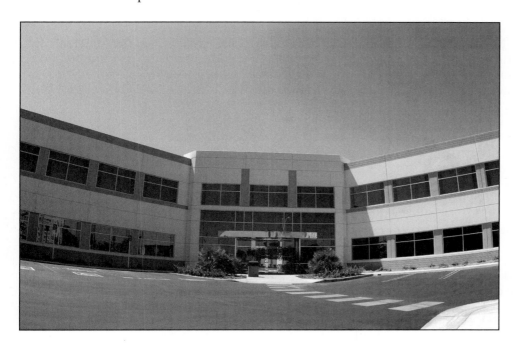

Figure P-4: South Padre Medical Center

The building houses several suites of professional offices. South Padre Medical Center is located in the middle of the building, just inside the front doors. The waiting room is the first area the patients enter. The front office area is separated from the patient waiting room by a registration desk. Figure P-5 shows Gladys at the registration desk.

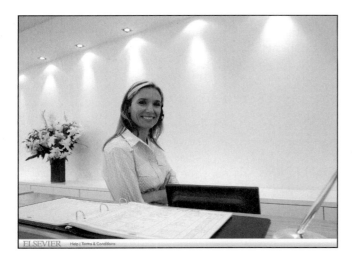

Figure P-5: Gladys Johnson at the South Padre Medical Center registration desk

A staff lounge is located at the rear of the Center, behind the laboratory area. The lounge is used by all employees for breaks throughout the day. There are picnic tables located outside the rear entrance for employee use. Smoking is not allowed within 100 feet of the center; thus there is no smoking at the picnic tables. Lockers are available in the lounge area, and all employees are required to place their personal items in a locker. Gladys Johnson, Medical Office Assistant, will assign you a locker and give you the combination to the lock. Personal items, such as purses and backpacks, are not allowed in the office area and must be stored in your locker at all times during your work day. Only medically necessary items are allowed in the office area. If you have medically necessary items, such as a nebulizer, please discuss this with Gladys before taking the items into the work area.

In consideration of our patients and employees with allergies and/or respiratory conditions, do not wear or apply perfumes, colognes, or other fragrances. Use only unscented hairsprays, deodorants, and other personal care items.

Each physician has a private office located a short distance from the patient examination rooms. When delivering mail or messages for the physicians, take them to the physician's private office. Never interrupt the physician in the patient examination rooms unless specifically told to do so by your supervisor or requested to do so by the physician.

A small laboratory is located in the Center; it is used for a variety of laboratory procedures. Staff members collect specimens, and some of the less complex analyses are conducted in the Center's laboratory by Center personnel. The Center has also contracted an outside laboratory, Island Express Labs, to do the Center's more complex specimen analysis. Each evening, a messenger from Island Express Labs delivers the results of previous analyses and picks up the specimens that are being sent out for analysis. Island Express Labs also returns results using the U.S. Postal Service.

Minor surgical procedures are sometimes conducted at the Center. The physicians are also on staff at South Padre Hospital, where they admit patients for more major surgeries. Procedures may be performed as either inpatient or outpatient procedures.

The South Padre Medical Complex building also houses offices of an independent radiologist; a psychiatrist; and an ear, nose, and throat (ENT) specialist. The physicians from the Center often refer patients to these physicians for consultation, and these physicians often refer patients to the physicians at the Center. You will be receiving patient information from these offices regarding patients that have been referred to the Center, and you will be sending patient information to these offices during your internship.

About Our Physicians

South Padre Medical Center was established to meet the health needs of South Padre residents in general/orthopedic surgery and family practice, with affiliates specializing in cardiology and surgery.

- **Dr. Gerald Bond**, a general and orthopedic surgeon, and **Dr. Ray Adams**, a family practitioner, founded the Center 20 years ago to provide health care to private patients and patients participating in Texas Health Corporation, a managed care organization.

- **Dr. Joyce Harkness**, a cardiologist, and **Dr. Anthony Clark**, a general surgeon, serve as affiliates to the Center. Dr. Harkness and Dr. Clark are from San Antonio and commute 2 days a week to see patients in the Center and at the hospital.

- All four physicians are registered with Texas Health Corporation as preferred providers. All physicians also have staff privileges at South Padre Hospital and South Padre Nursing Home.

PRE-TASK **1.4**

SOFTWARE ORIENTATION

Many terms can be used to describe the computerized storage of patient medical information—for instance, CPR (computerized patient record), EHR (electronic health record), and EMR (electronic medical record). Each term has in common the fact that the medical documentation is maintained in an electronic environment. Some electronic record systems simply scan old paper documents into a new electronic record. The scanning method is usually used when facilities begin the transition from a paper to an electronic system (historical patient information is scanned into the new electronic record).

In 1996, national standards for health care information were set in the Federal Health Insurance Portability and Accountability Act (HIPAA), and in 2003 a Privacy Rule was enacted that addressed the transmissions of electronic health documents. Today, HIPAA regulates the maintenance and transmittal of medical records that are in an electronic format.

Many facilities are now in transition to the electronic format because of the many cost-saving and communication advantages to using an EHR system. Communication about patient care is enhanced with a single, life-long electronic health record for a patient, and a central record reduces the potential for errors when providing health care to a patient and recording information about the patient. The eventual goal is to have a single patient health record for every patient in the country. When this goal is achieved, every health care provider will access the patient record electronically and all information about the patient's health care will be in one central location that is globally accessible.

Currently, a single, set standard does not exist to capture, store, and access the electronic data in a facility; rather, private companies have developed a variety of proprietary software systems. Each system has different features, functions, and capabilities, but in general, they all store patient health information. You can be assured that an electronic health record system will be part of every medical facility in the future. You will be using the MedTrak system, which is excellent EHR software and very typical of what you will encounter on the job.

Software Introduction

The push for the EHR is necessitated by the Centers for Medicare and Medicaid Services (CMS) as a cost-cutting measure. Since the federal government is the largest third-party payer in the country, it is critical that health care providers follow the guidelines established by the government. The CMS mandate for electronic health records is a nonfunded mandate, which means that medical facilities have to purchase, install, and implement an EHR system at their own expense. Some federal funds have been appropriated to help smaller practices make the transition, but the majority of the costs are the responsibility of the facility. Larger medical facilities have been first to implement an EHR system, with the majority of smaller physician practices just now in the process of adopting a system.

For this project, you will be using MedTrak's web-based software, which combines the EHR with practice management. Practice management software enables the provider to complete a wide variety of daily office tasks using a system that is integrated with the EHR. For example, when preparing a bill for a patient, the software will access the patient's address and account information all at one time; this differs from other types of software where the patient information is in one system and the accounting information is in another system. **MedTrak is designed to work best with Internet Explorer, version 6.0 or newer.**

Task 1-2 will be your overview of the capabilities and functions of the software. The remainder of the tasks in Days 1 through 10 are the practical application of these functions.

You will log on to the MedTrak website directly through the South Padre Medical Center/MedTrak Systems link on the companion Evolve site. The work that you do in the EHR environment will be saved so that the next time you return to the site to continue your work, your previous work will be there. For example, if you change information in a patient's medical record, the updated information will be displayed the next time you access that patient's record. Since each task builds upon the previous task, please complete the tasks in the order in which they are presented.

The activities have been created in a step-by-step format that makes learning simple. Just follow the directions, and by the time you are finished with this manual you will know how to maneuver through an EHR like a professional.

You need this workbook and the following to begin:

1. Access to the Internet with Internet Explorer, version 6.0 or newer
2. Your Course ID number, provided by your instructor

You are ready to learn something new and exciting, so let's begin by logging on to the Evolve website and enrolling in the course.

Evolve Course Enrollment

Visit http://evolve.elsevier.com/enroll. Enter the Course ID number (provided by your instructor) in the field provided.

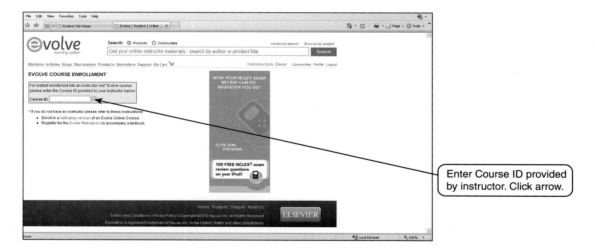

Verify that the course information is correct. Select the **Yes, this is my course** check box. Select the "I already have an access code:" radio button. Type the access code (see inside front cover of this student manual) into the text box and click **Register**.

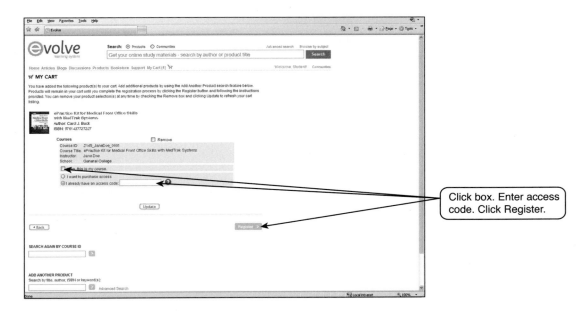

Click box. Enter access code. Click Register.

If you already have an Evolve account or have previously requested products from Evolve, provide your case-sensitive username and password in the Returning User area and click **Login**. If you do not have an Evolve account, provide your desired password for the account in the New User area and click **Continue**. Provide the required profile information and click **Continue**.

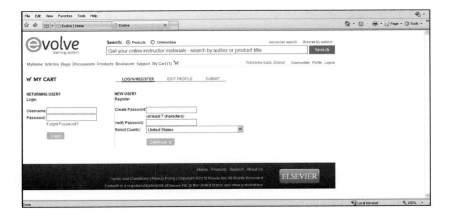

After your username and password have been accepted, read and accept the Registered User Agreement. Then click the box for **Yes, I accept this agreement** and click the **Submit** button.

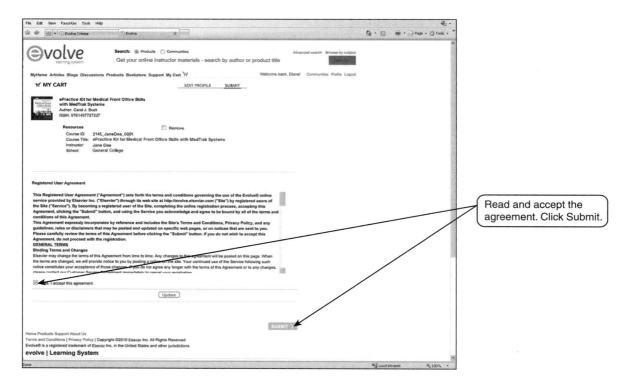

After a short period, confirmation of your enrollment will appear. An e-mail is then sent to the course instructor(s) and to your e-mail as well. The message sent to you will contain your Evolve account information, including username and password. You may then click the **Get Started!** link.

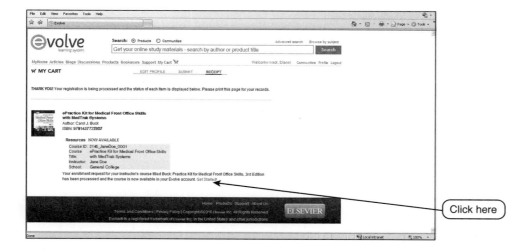

This is an example of the e-mail you will receive.

Doe, John

From: evolve-admin@elsevier.com
Sent: Current Date, Current Time
To: Doe, John (ELS-STL)
Subject: Evolve Student Self-Enrollment into Instructor-led Course.

Dear John Doe,

You have been enrolled in Buck: ePractice Kit for Medical Front Office Skills with MedTrak Systems. If you have any questions or problems related to the course, please contact your instructor.

The course is located in your Evolve account:

Username: jdoe
Password: evolve1

<u>Click here</u> to log in.

Welcome to Evolve!

Visit the <u>Evolve Support Portal</u> to access the Evolve Knowledge Base, Downloads, and Support Ticket system. Live Evolve Support is also available by calling 1-800-401-9962, 24 hours 7 days a week.

Copyright © 2012 Elsevier Inc. All Rights Reserved. Evolve® is a registered trademark of <u>Elsevier Inc.</u> in the United States and other jurisdictions. <u>Home</u> | <u>Privacy Policy</u> | <u>Terms and Conditions</u>

After you click the **Get Started!** button on the Receipt/Registration Confirmation page, you will see the page below. On the top left side of the page, under Resources, you will see the book title, course ID, and instructor name listed. To access the Resources, click on the book title.

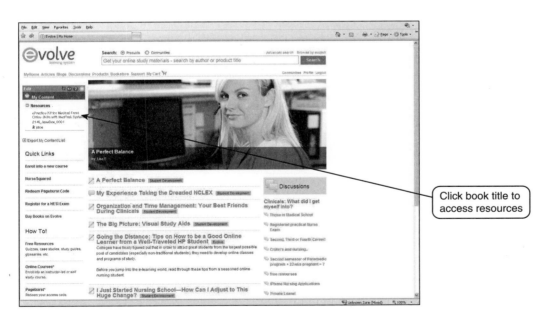

Click book title to access resources

The next page shows the name of the book, as well as grade information. Click on **Start this course at the beginning**.

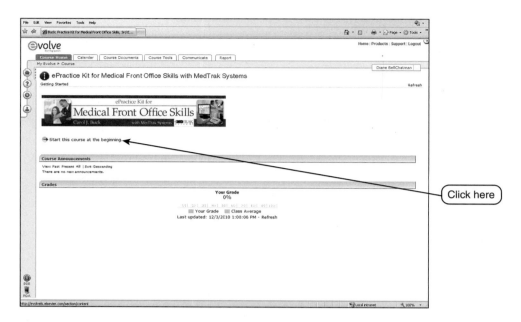

The Course Documents page shows the Resources and South Padre Medical Center/MedTrak Systems links. Click on the **Resources** link to access your Evolve Resources. Click on the **South Padre Medical Center/MedTrak Systems** link to access the MedTrak program.

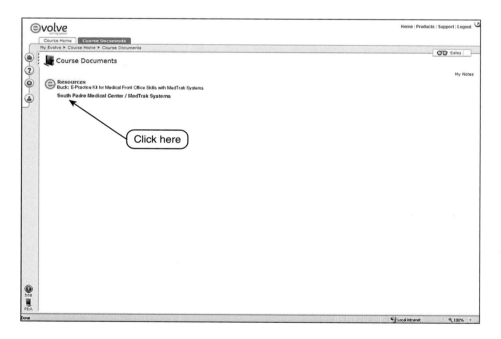

The first time you enter MedTrak, you will see the screen below. Enter your initials and full name in the spaces provided and click **Submit**. This screen will only appear the first time you enter MedTrak. The next time you log in, you will be taken straight to the MedTrak Main Menu.

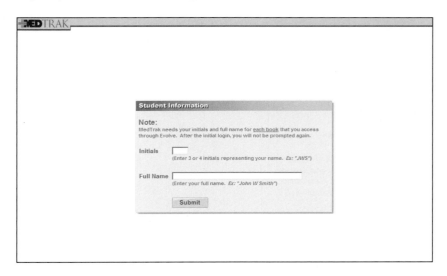

You are responsible for ensuring that no one has access to your Evolve login information. If your access information is compromised, immediately notify your instructor. You may obtain technical assistance on the functionality of Evolve and MedTrak by contacting Elsevier Support at 800-401-9962.

Now that you are enrolled in Evolve, the screen shown below is where you will type in your login information every time you log in to Evolve. You can access this screen by typing http://evolve.elsevier.com in your browser.

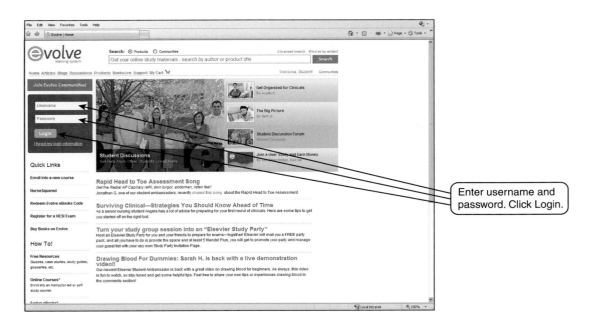

Main Menu

The Main Menu of the software is called the Dashboard, as illustrated in Figure P-6.

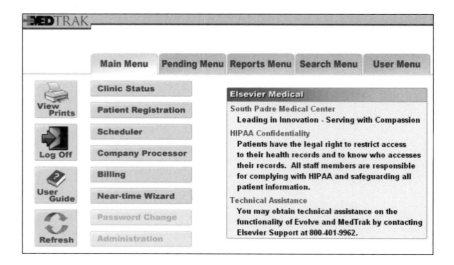

Figure P-6: Main Dashboard of the software

Let's begin at the Main Menu and learn about some of the key functions of this software. When the software launches, the Main Menu tab is displayed on the main Dashboard with buttons for the following available functions:

1. Center Status
2. Patient Registration
3. Scheduler
4. Company Processor
5. Billing
6. Near-time Wizard

Clinic Status

Click on the **Clinic Status** button (illustrated in Figure P-7).

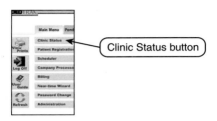

Figure P-7: Clinic Status button on the Dashboard

The Clinic Status screen opens, as displayed in Figure P-8.

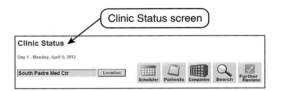

Figure P-8: Clinic Status screen

Displayed is the name of the screen (Clinic Status), followed by the day of the internship, in "month, day, year" format. The date displayed on your screen is the day of the internship. For example, note in Figure P-8 that the date in red following the Clinic Status is Day 1—Monday, April 9, 2012, indicating that this is the first day of your internship. The yellow highlighting on the computer screen indicates the active field. Also, note that in Figure P-8 the active field is the Location, which in this case is South Padre Medical Center.

Caution: Each time you access a screen, you leave a digital footprint, which is a history trail your supervisor may review to determine the information you have viewed. Only access information that you are authorized to access to complete your tasks.

Exercise P-1

Active Field

1. What field is active in Figure P-8, the Clinic Status screen?
   a. There is no active field
   b. Clinic Status
   c. Location
   d. CMD

2. How did you determine which field was active on the screen?
   a. The field was blank
   b. The field was highlighted
   c. There is no way to determine whether the field is active
   d. There are multiple active fields on each screen at one time

If the facility had multiple locations, such as several centers or multiple divisions within one center, the location could be changed by clicking the **Location** button, as illustrated in Figure P-9. For our purposes, the Location button will be used to display the different physicians who practice at the South Padre Medical Center.

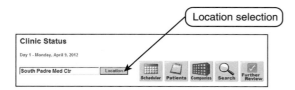

Figure P-9: Multiple location selection

Click the **Location** button now, and the screen shown in Figure P-10 will display a list of available physicians.

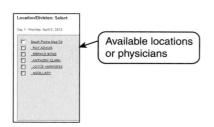

Figure P-10: Available locations or physicians

Next, click the **Exit Screen** button twice, as illustrated in Figure P-11, to return to the Clinic Status screen. On some screens, MedTrak requires clicking **Exit Screen** twice to ensure that you really meant to exit the screen.

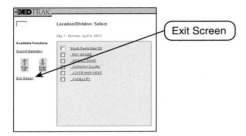

Figure P-11: Exit Screen button

Develop the habit of clicking the **Exit Screen** button instead of using the back arrow on your Internet browser. The software is designed to return to the correct screen only when the Exit Screen link is used. Once back on the Clinic Status screen, let's continue learning about the Available Functions on the left side of the screen:

1. Submit/Refresh
2. Name/Reason
3. Nursing Notes
4. Examine Patient
5. Order Entry
6. Open Orders
7. Provider's Notes
8. Out The Door
9. Discharge
10. Done
11. Schedule
12. Visit Log
13. Online Chart
14. View Prints
15. More Functions

Place your cursor in the CMD (Command) box, as illustrated in Figure P-12, and click the left button on your mouse. The CMD field is now active, which means that the software is waiting for a command to be placed in the box. You can change the highlighted area by clicking in another CMD box. Place your cursor in another CMD box, and note that the newly selected box is highlighted in yellow, meaning the box is now active.

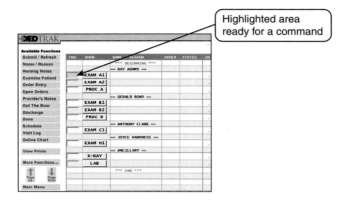

Figure P-12: Highlighted box is the active box

It is from the Clinic Status screen that the first step in management of patient data begins. The Available Functions buttons on the left of the screen allow you to access the various features of the software. Let's perform an exercise that will require you to click into various Available Function buttons determine the display for each function.

Exercise P-2

Available Functions

Place your cursor in the Command box next to "Exam A1" and left-click your mouse to highlight the box. Match each Available Function button to the information that appears in the highlighted CMD box when you click that button. For example, when you click the **Examine Patient** button, EXPT appears in the highlighted CMD box. Answers in the Displayed in the CMD Box column may be used more than once.

Available Function Button

1. _____ Submit/Refresh
2. _____ Name/Reason
3. _____ Nursing Notes
4. _____ Examine Patient
5. _____ Order Entry
6. _____ Open Orders
7. _____ Provider's Notes
8. _____ Out The Door
9. _____ Discharge
10. _____ Done
11. _____ Schedule
12. _____ Visit Log
13. _____ Online Chart
14. _____ View Prints
15. _____ More Functions

Displayed in the CMD Box

a. EXPT

b. DIS

c. OPENS TO THE SCHEDULING SCREEN

d. NN

e. OTD

f. O

g. CHRT

h. OPENS TO SCREEN DISPLAYING ADDITIONAL FUNCTIONS AS IN FIGURE P-13

i. CL

j. X

k. DONE

l. OPENS TO AVAILABLE USER REPORT

m. NOTHING HAPPENS WITHOUT A PATIENT NAME PREVIOUSLY ENTERED

n. OTD

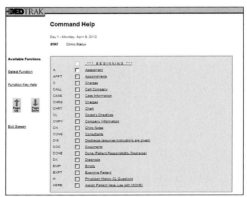

Figure P-13: Command Help screen

Patient Database

Great job! You are making good progress on this new EHR information. Now let's start using these functions with patient information. To begin, click on the **Patients** button on the top of the Clinic Status screen, as illustrated in Figure P-14.

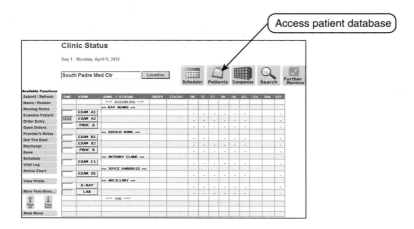

Figure P-14: Accessing the patient database

The alphabetically ordered patient database is displayed in Figure P-15.

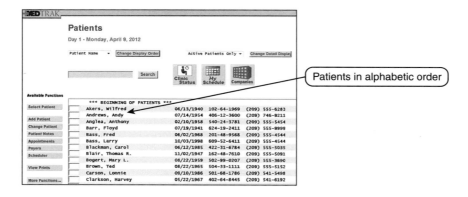

Figure P-15: Patients in alphabetic order in the database

The order in which the patients in the database are displayed can be changed by clicking the drop-down arrow next to Patient Name, as shown in Figure P-16.

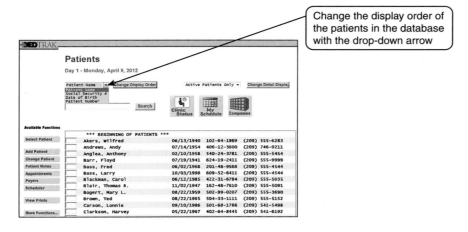

Figure P-16: Changing of the display of the patients in the database

The patient database can be viewed in order of Social Security number, date of birth, or patient number. On the Patients screen, click the drop-down arrow next to Patient Name and highlight **Social Security #** on the drop-down menu. Then click the **Change Display Order** button to the right of the drop-down arrow.

When you do this, the patient data will appear by Social Security number in descending order, as illustrated in Figure P-17.

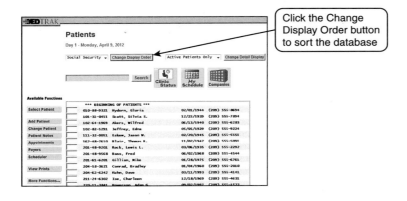

Figure P-17: Sorting the patient database

Exercise P-3

Sorting the Patient Database

Answer the following questions about sorting the patient database:

1. When you sort the patient database by Social Security number, who is the fourth patient listed in the database? _____

2. When you sort the patient database by date of birth, what is the telephone number of the first patient listed? _____

The patient database can also be sorted according to the patient's status. Figure P-18 illustrates the use of the Change Detail Display drop-down arrow to display patient data based on the patient classification of:

- Active Patients Only
- Deleted Patients Only
- All Patients (both active and deleted—all patients in database)

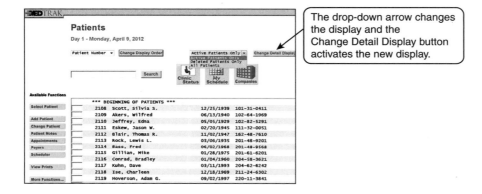

Figure P-18: Change Detail Display drop-down arrow

Note the Search box in Figure P-19, in which you can enter a patient name, patient number, Social Security number, or date of birth to locate patients.

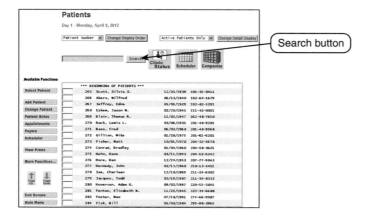

Figure P-19: Patient Search button

Now let's use the various features you have just learned about by completing another exercise.

Exercise P-4

Patient Search

Answer the following questions about sorting the patient database using both the Change Detail Display and the Change Display Order drop-down arrow:

1. Set the display (remember to click the button to the right of the drop-down arrow to activate your selection) to Active Patients Only by Social Security #. Then identify the patient whose Social Security number is 162-48-7610. _____

2. Set the display to All Patients by Date of Birth. Then identify the patient with the birthdate of 03/06/1935. _____

3. With the display set to Active Patients by Patient Name, type the name "Lorenz" in the Search box. Then click the **Search** button or hit **ENTER** on your keyboard. What is Ms. Lorenz's first name? _____

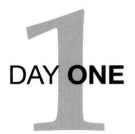

DAY ONE

Monday, April 9, 2012

TASK **1.1**	Preparing the Schedules
TASK **1.2**	Scheduling Walk-Ins and Surgeries
TASK **1.3**	Entering Patient Data

TASK **1.1**

PREPARING THE SCHEDULES

 Requirements

- Access to the physicians' schedules using MedTrak

Gladys has asked you to prepare (matrix) the schedule for two weeks in November by blocking off the times when the physicians will not be available. Gladys will prepare the schedule prior to November 11. You will begin by matrixing the schedule for Dr. Bond for November 12-23, 2012.

November 2012

Sun	Mon	Tue	Wed	Thur	Fri	Sat
				1	2	3
4	5	6	7	8	9	10
11	12	13	14	15	16	17
18	19	20	21	22	23	24
25	26	27	28	29	30	

Figure 1-1: November 2012 calendar

Locations

Log on to MedTrak through the Evolve website. From the main Dashboard, click the **Clinic Status** button that you learned about earlier. Then click the **Location** button to the right of the Location field to display the location choices. Place your cursor in the box next to Dr. Bond's name and click the **Submit Selection** link to the left of the box located above the green arrows (as shown in Figure 1-2).

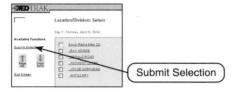

Figure 1-2: Submit Selection link on the left side of the screen

Scheduling Screen

Dr. Bond's Clinic Status page is then displayed, as illustrated in Figure 1-3.

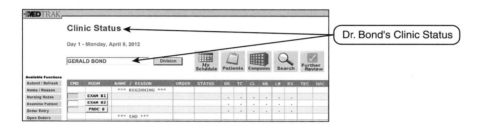

Figure 1-3: Dr. Bond's Clinic Status screen

In the list of Available Functions, click **Schedule**, as shown in Figure 1-4, to display Dr. Bond's schedule.

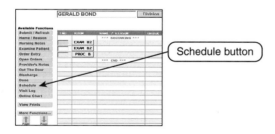

Figure 1-4: Dr. Bond's schedule

Dr. Bond's schedule will be displayed with the yellow (active) box at 8:00a, as in Figure 1-5.

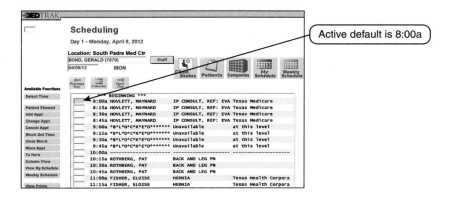

Figure 1-5: Dr. Bond's scheduling screen

To complete your assignment from Gladys to matrix two weeks in November, you will need to display Dr. Bond's November schedule. To do this, click the **Calendar** button located below the date on the Schedule screen, as illustrated in Figure 1-6.

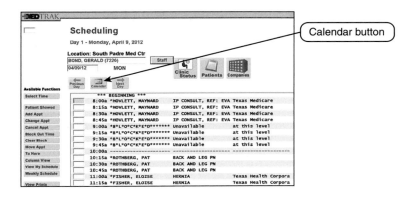

Figure 1-6: Calendar button

After clicking the **Calendar** button, the screen will display the month of April 2012, as shown in Figure 1-7. From this screen, click the **Next Month** right arrow until you reach November 2012. You can return to April 2012 by clicking the **Last Month** blue arrow on the left side of the calendar. If you have moved your calendar view to November, return to April 2012.

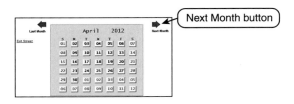

Figure 1-7: Current monthly calendar

Once you are back on the April 2012 monthly calendar, click on **April 9, 2012**, to learn about another way to access a future date. From the April 9, 2012, scheduling screen, enter "11/12/12" in the date field (Figure 1-8) and click **ENTER** on your keyboard.

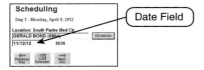

Figure 1-8: Date field

The Scheduling screen will then display the day schedule for 11/12/12. You can then click **Calendar**, and the screen will display the month of November, as illustrated in Figure 1-9. In the monthly view, you can click on any day and display the schedule for that day.

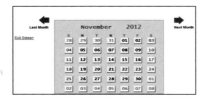

Figure 1-9: November 2012 displayed on Calendar screen

To complete the next step, you must have 11/12/12 displayed on Dr. Bond's Scheduling screen. You can accomplish this either by clicking the **Next Month** arrow on the Calendar screen or by entering the date in the date field.

Click **12** on the November calendar to display the schedule for Monday, November 12, 2012, as illustrated in Figure 1-10.

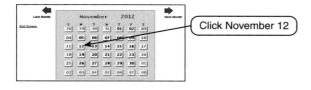

Figure 1-10: Accessing a day of the month

The cursor will already be highlighting the 8:00a block, which is the default block. To ensure you are on the correct date, verify that the date field displays 11/12/12.

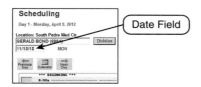

Figure 1-11: Date field indicates schedule date displayed on the screen

Blocking (Matrixing)

With your screen displaying the date 11/12/12, click **Block Out Time** on the left, as illustrated in Figure 1-12.

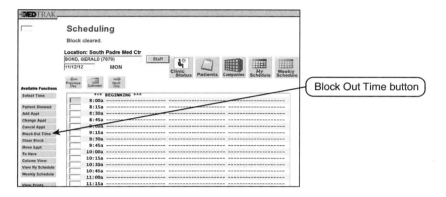

Figure 1-12: Block Out Time button

The screen will display the block-out feature, as illustrated in Figure 1-13. The fields indicate the beginning and ending time of the block-out. For now, click the **Exit Screen** link on left side of the screen twice to return to Dr. Bond's main scheduling screen.

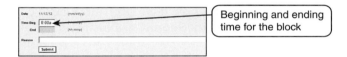

Figure 1-13: Blocking out time on the Scheduling screen

If you enter blocking incorrectly, place your cursor next to any time within the blocked time and click **Clear Block** (located under **Block**) and a box will be displayed to confirm that you want to remove the blocking, as illustrated in Figure 1-14.

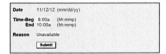

Figure 1-14: Clearing blocking

You are now ready to begin matrixing the schedule. Matrix Dr. Bond's schedule first. Dr. Bond's office hours are as follows:

Monday	Tuesday	Wednesday	Thursday	Friday
10-6	9-5	9-12	9-12	8-5

Unavailable Times

Dr. Bond has requested not to be scheduled in the office before 10 a.m. on Monday. Block the time from 8-10 a.m., entering "Unavailable" as the reason, as shown in Figure 1-15.

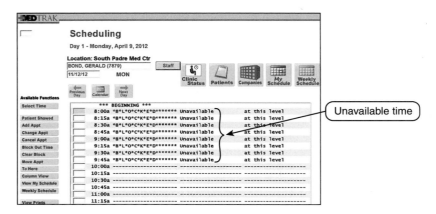

Figure 1-15: Matrixing time as unavailable

Use "a" to denote "a.m." and "p" to denote "p.m." Note that the format for entering the time is hh:mm (hourhour:minuteminute); therefore you will either add a zero before any three-digit time block (for example, type 01:00p) or hit the space bar to leave a blank space before the first digit in a three-digit time (for example, hit space bar and then type 1:00p). When you have the correct times entered, click **Submit**, as illustrated in Figure 1-16, to complete the blocking process.

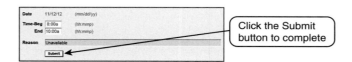

Figure 1-16: Completing the blocking process

Block the same time period (8-10 a.m.) on Dr. Bond's Monday, November 19, 2012, schedule.

Lunch Hours

Lunch is one hour in length for all physicians and is scheduled from 12-1 p.m. on days when the physician's office hours begin at 8 a.m. or 9 a.m. and from 1-2 p.m. when the office hours begin at 10 a.m. To block off the lunch hour, first place your cursor in the box next to the time that the lunch hour begins; once the box is highlighted, click **Block Out Time**. Enter "Lunch" as the Reason.

To view times after 12:00 p.m., click the green **Page Down** arrow until the desired time is reached (illustrated in Figure 1-17).

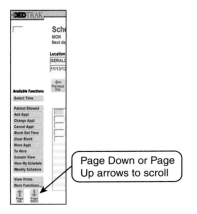

Figure 1-17: Viewing schedule after 12:00 p.m.

Click the green **Page Down** arrow once more to view Dr. Bond's schedule for late afternoon. Figure 1-18 displays Dr. Bond's afternoon schedule.

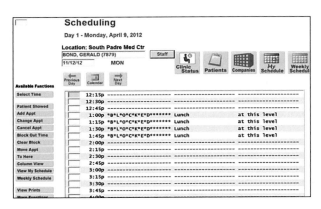

Figure 1-18: Dr. Bond's matrixed lunch hours for 11/12/12

Dr. Bond's lunch hours for the week are:

Monday	Tuesday	Wednesday	Thursday	Friday
1-2	12-1	12-1	12-1	12-1

Block the lunch hours for Dr. Bond for 11/12/2012-11/23/2012.

End-of-Day

You must also mark off any time periods at the end of the day that Dr. Bond has indicated are not to be scheduled. Dr. Bond wants to complete his schedule no later than 5 p.m. on Tuesdays; therefore you would mark off the four 15-minute time blocks from 5 p.m. to 6 p.m., as shown in Figure 1-19.

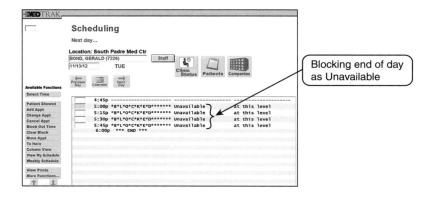

Figure 1-19: Blocking end of day as Unavailable

Block the following time periods at the end of the day as Unavailable:

Monday	Tuesday	Wednesday	Thursday	Friday
None	5-6 pm	4-6 pm	4-6 pm	5-6 pm

Rounds

Dr. Bond conducts inpatient rounds from 6 a.m. to 8:45 a.m. on Tuesdays and Wednesdays. Mark off his schedule from 8-8:45 a.m. as "Rounds" and from 8:45-9:00 a.m. as "Travel" to allow travel time from the hospital to the Center, as illustrated in Figure 1-20.

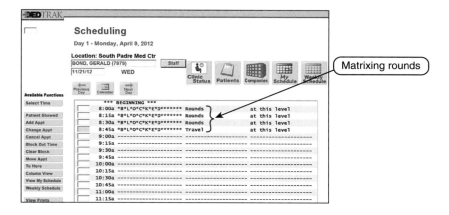

Figure 1-20: Dr. Bond's rounds and travel matrixed on the schedule

Board Meetings

Dr. Bond also has a board meeting each Thursday from 7:30-8:45 a.m., as shown in Figure 1-21. You will also schedule 15 additional minutes of travel time after the meeting to allow him time to return to the center.

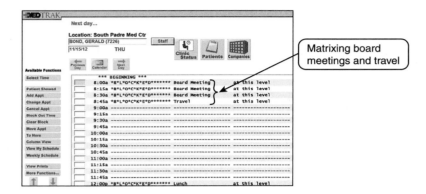

Figure 1-21: Dr. Bond's board meeting and travel scheduled on Thursdays

Mark off Dr. Bond's board meetings for 11/12/2012-11/23/2012.

Surgery Schedule

Dr. Bond has reserved Wednesday and Thursday from 1-4 p.m. for his surgery schedule. On these days, Dr. Bond has a lunch break from 12-1 p.m.; he also uses that time to travel the 15 minutes to the hospital, so no additional travel time needs to be scheduled and travel does not need to be indicated on the schedule. Figure 1-22 illustrates Dr. Bond's surgery schedule.

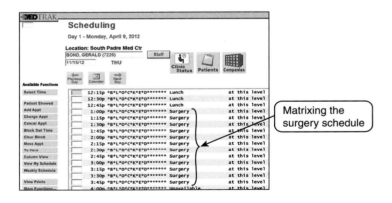

Figure 1-22: Dr. Bond's surgery schedule

Block off Dr. Bond's surgery schedule for 11/12/2012-11/23/2012.

Schedule Printing

You have blocked off all 10 days of Dr. Bond's schedule for 11/12/2012-11/23/2012, and it is time to print the schedule. Click **More Functions** located just above the green arrows on the lower left of the page; the screen will be displayed as in Figure 1-23.

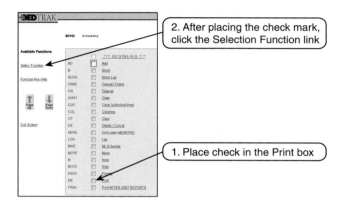

Figure 1-23: Print accessed through the More Functions button

To access the screen illustrated in Figure 1-24, place a check mark in the Print box and then **Select Function**.

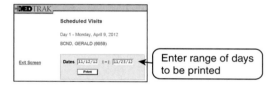

Figure 1-24: Select schedule dates to print

Enter 11/12/12-11/23/12 as the dates of the schedule to print; then click the **Print** button. When you click **Print**, the schedule is printed to a report in PDF format. The message "Report sent to the printer ..." will appear at the top of the screen under the screen title. To view the report that you have created, click the **Exit Screen** button on the left of the screen to return to Dr. Bond's main screen.

Click **View Prints** on the lower left side of the screen, as illustrated in Figure 1-25.

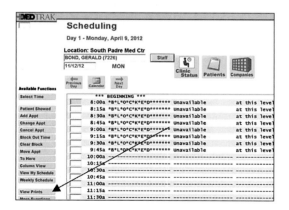

Figure 1-25: View Prints button (Dr. Bond's schedule)

The View Prints screen will open, and a new window displays the reports that are ready in the Available User Reports area; see Figure 1-26.

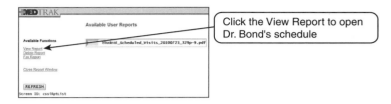

Click the View Report to open Dr. Bond's schedule

Figure 1-26: Available User Reports window

The default is the report you just created, so all you need do is click **View Report** and the report will be displayed, as shown in Figure 1-27. Click the printer icon on the toolbar to print the pages of the report for Dr. Bond. You should have two pages of schedules printed for Dr. Bond for the time period of 11/12/2012-11/23/2012.

Print the schedule

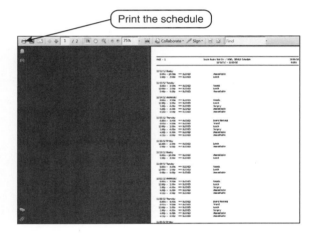

Figure 1-27: Viewing and printing the report

Next, you will save the schedule you just printed.

Saving Completed Work

Save Dr. Bond's schedule in the Day 1, Task 1.1 subfolder of your Completed Work folder as LastName_ YourFirstInitial_Task1.1Bond.pdf. To save a document, click the save icon on the toolbar (Figure 1-28).

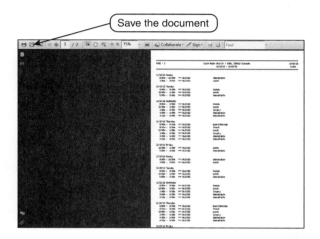

Figure 1-28: Save icon on PDF report

In the **Save a Copy** window, select the location where your Completed Work folder is located, as shown in Figure 1-29.

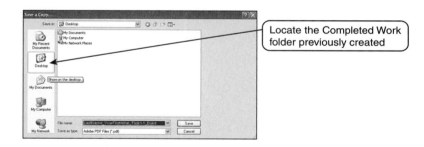

Figure 1-29: Saving to your Completed Work folder

Double-click the Completed Work folder as shown in Figure 1-30. Name the document using this format: LastName_YourFirstInitial_Task1.1_Bond.pdf.

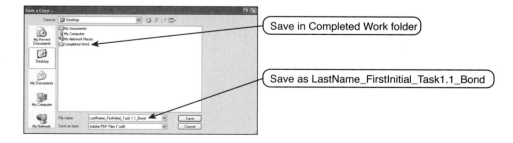

Figure 1-30: Saving to your Completed Work folder

Matrixing for Other Physicians

It is now time to matrix the 11/12/2012-11/23/2012 schedule for the other physicians. Refer to the directions for Dr. Bond's schedule if you have questions about how to complete the matrixing.

Physician Schedule	Monday	Tuesday	Wednesday	Thursday	Friday
Dr. Ray Adams	9-6	9-6	10-5	9-12	9-5
Dr. Joyce Harkness	None	None	2-6	2-6	None
Dr. Anthony Clark	None	None	2-6	2-6	None

- Lunch breaks for all physicians are 1 hour in length and are scheduled from 12-1 p.m. for physicians on days when the office hours begin at 8 a.m. or 9 a.m.; when office hours begin at 10 a.m., lunch breaks are scheduled from 1-2 p.m.

Physician Preferences

Dr. Ray Adams

1. Board meeting the third Wednesday of each month from 8-9:45 a.m., with 15 minutes additional travel time to the center indicated on the schedule. The board meeting does not affect Dr. Adams' lunch schedule, since his office hours remain the same.
2. Rounds on Monday, Thursday, and Friday from 7-8:45 a.m. with 15 minutes travel time.
3. Teaches a class at the local medical school (note as "Medical School") from 1-3 p.m. each Thursday. Although he has lunch from noon to 1 p.m. on this day, he requests that you indicate "Travel" on his schedule from 12:30-1 p.m. as a reminder. Dr. Adams does not return to the office after the class if he has finished his clinical work. Block off his time from 3 p.m. and after as "Unavailable."
4. Block off any times before or after the scheduled times as "Unavailable." For example, on Tuesday, block off the hour between 8 and 9 a.m. because Dr. Adams schedule does not begin until 9 a.m. that day.
5. Print Dr. Adams' schedule for 11/12/2012-11/23/2012.

Dr. Anthony Clark and Dr. Joyce Harkness

1. Rounds on Wednesday and Thursday from 8-9 a.m. with no travel time after because the physicians do not travel back to the center, but instead begin surgery at the hospital.
2. Surgery from 9 a.m. to 1 p.m. on Wednesdays and Thursdays.
3. Lunch from 1-2 p.m. on Wednesdays and Thursdays.
4. Leave the period from 2-6 p.m. blank; this is when the physicians return to the center to attend to their scheduled patients. No travel time is necessary on either day for either physician.
5. Print the schedules for both Dr. Clark and Dr. Harkness for 11/12/2012-11/23/2012.

Print the schedules for Drs. Adams, Clark, and Harkness. Save each report in your Completed Work folder as you did Dr. Bond's schedule, using the naming conventions below.

Physician	File Name
Dr. Ray Adams	LastName_YourFirstInitial_Task1.1Adams
Dr. Joyce Harkness	LastName_YourFirstInitial_Task1.1Harkness
Dr. Anthony Clark	LastName_YourFirstInitial_Task1.1Clark

When you have saved all of your reports for Task 1.1 to your Completed Work folder, delete them by placing the cursor in the box beside each report and clicking **Delete Report** on the left side of the screen (Figure 1-31). A pop-up box will appear to ask whether you are certain you want to delete the report. Click **OK**. Do this for each one of the reports you generated, so that the queue is empty when you begin Task 1.2.

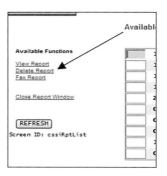

Figure 1-31: Deleting reports

Task **1.2**

SCHEDULING WALK-INS AND SURGERIES

Scheduling Walk-Ins

It is now 9:50 a.m. and Kathy Forest, a patient of Dr. Adams, comes into the center and walks to the reception desk where you and Gladys are working. Kathy says that she has a "terrible headache and a little fever" and would like to see Dr. Adams if he is available. Gladys tells the patient that Dr. Adams can see her in about 10 minutes, asks the patient to be seated in the waiting room, and then assists you with scheduling the appointment. Gladys asks you to register Kathy for a 10 a.m. appointment with Dr. Adams. You are to check the appointment scheduling guidelines for the appropriate length of time for the appointment (located at the end of this chapter and in Appendix A).

From the Clinic Status screen, change the Location to Dr. Adams, and on the left side of the screen open his schedule. Your screen should display as shown in Figure 1-32.

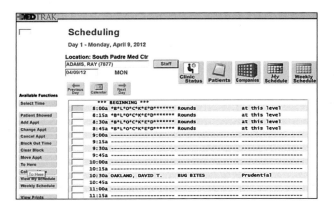

Figure 1-32: Schedule screen for Dr. Adams for 04/09/12

To schedule Kathy for the 10:00a appointment time, highlight that time and click **Add Appt** on the left side of screen, as shown in Figure 1-33. This will open the patient database.

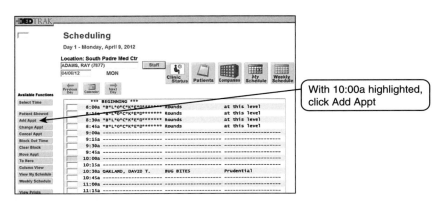

Figure 1-33: Adding an appointment

Locate Kathy Forest's name from the patient database, and place your cursor in the box next to the name to highlight the box. Click **Select** on the left side of the screen, as displayed in Figure 1-34.

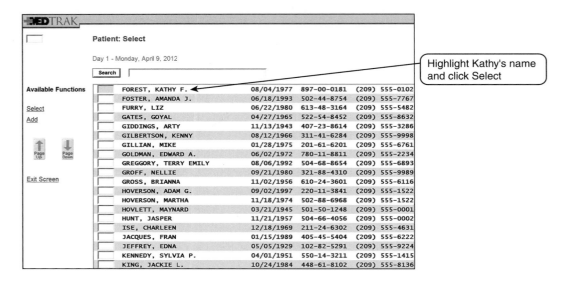

Figure 1-34: Select Kathy F. Forest's name

When you click **Select**, you are directed to the screen to confirm the payer. Kathy is a self-pay patient, which is her default, so click the **Confirm Payer** button on the left, as shown in Figure 1-35.

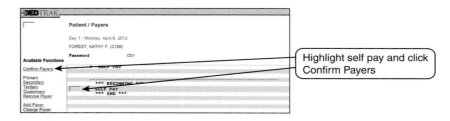

Figure 1-35: Confirming the payer

On the next screen, you will record the appointment length and the reason for the appointment, as illustrated in Figure 1-36. The reason is "Headache/Fever," and according to the appointment scheduling guidelines located at the end of this text, the length of the appointment is 30 minutes. After entering this information, click **Submit** at the bottom of the dialog box.

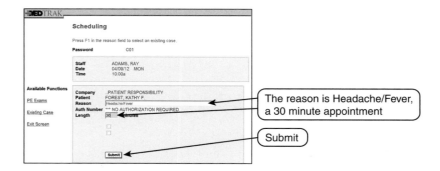

Figure 1-36: Entering the reason and length of the appointment

When you click **Submit**, a screen to enter any additional notes is displayed. Since there are no further notes for Kathy, type "None" in the shaded area and click **Submit Note** on the left side of the screen, as shown in Figure 1-37.

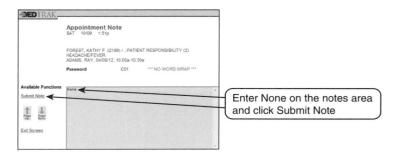

Figure 1-37: Completing the note

After you click **Submit Note**, you are returned to Dr. Adams' scheduling screen, which shows Kathy Forest's appointment as scheduled, as illustrated in Figure 1-38.

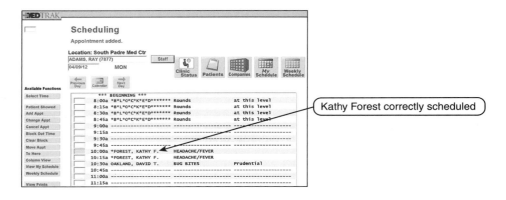

Figure 1-38: Kathy Forest's appointment scheduled

Using the directions provided earlier for saving a copy of the schedule, save a copy of Dr. Adams' schedule for 04/09/12, and place it in your Completed Work folder in the Day 1, Task 1.2 subfolder.

- Save the document as LastName_YourFirstInitial_Task1.2Adams

Good Job! You completed this appointment like a real professional! Gladys is pleased with how quickly you are learning to operate the MedTrak software.

Now Gladys tells you that Dr. Bond has decided to take this afternoon off and catch up with some paperwork at the hospital. He has asked that his schedule after lunch until 6 p.m. be noted as "Unavailable." Gladys asks you to block Dr. Bond's schedule for the time indicated following the directions she gave you earlier on blocking. Once you have blocked Dr. Bond's time, save a copy of Dr. Bond's schedule for 04/09/12 and place it in your Completed Work folder in Day 1, Task 1.2 subfolder.

- Save the document as LastName_YourFirstInitial_Task1.2Bond09

Dr. Adams has asked that you schedule Jackie W. Masci with Dr. Clark for a 2:45 p.m. appointment on 04/12/12 for a breast mass. Note on Jackie's appointment that Dr. Adams referred this patient (Ref Adams) to Dr. Clark. Once you have scheduled the appointment, use the directions provided earlier to save a copy of Dr. Clark's schedule for 04/12/12 and place it in your Completed Work folder in Day 1, Task 1.2 subfolder.

- Save the document as LastName_YourFirstInitial_Task1.2Clark12

Scheduling Surgery

The morning is going quickly, and Gladys wants you to schedule four surgeries. Three of the these are for Dr. Bond's patients and one is for Dr. Adams' patient. Gladys has made notes of how these surgeries are to be scheduled but wants you to input the information in the schedules for the physicians. Obtain the length of surgery from the appointment scheduling guidelines at the end of this chapter. Recall that the surgical schedules have been blocked, so you are to clear the blocking, enter the patient on the schedule, and then reblock the remainder of the time that was previously blocked so others do not schedule office visits during the surgical times. For example, let's say that Dr. Bond's schedule was blocked for 3 hours of surgery time and you remove the blocking and schedule a 1-hour surgical procedure. You then need to reblock the other 2 hours of the surgery schedule.

Dr. Bond's directions:

1. Eloise Fisher, schedule at 1 p.m., 04/11/12, for inguinal hernia repair.
2. Carol Smith, schedule at 3 p.m., 04/12/12, for a microdiscectomy.
3. Terry Emily Greggory, schedule at 1 p.m., 04/12/12, for an L4/L5 laminectomy.

Dr. Adams' directions:

1. William J. Foley, schedule with Dr. Clark at 9 a.m., 04/18/12, for an inguinal hernia repair.

Using the directions provided earlier on printing and saving a copy of the physician's schedule, save a copy of Dr. Bond's schedule for 04/11/12 and 04/12/12 and place it in your Completed Work folder in the Day 1, Task 1.2 subfolder.

For Dr. Bond, you will have two days to save; one for 04/11/12 and one for 04/12/12.

- Save the 04/11/12 document as LastName_YourFirstInitial_Task1.2Bond11
- Save the 04/12/12 document as LastName_YourFirstInitial_Task1.2Bond12

If you print Dr. Bond's schedule from 04/11/12-04/12/12, you will get a weekly schedule (see Figure 1-39), such as the one you printed for him after you blocked his November schedule. However, instead of that weekly schedule, you are now to save a daily schedule, which requires you to save each day separately. Figures 1-40 and 1-41 illustrate the correct result of saving Dr. Bond's schedule one day at a time.

```
=================================================================================================
PAGE - 1                       South Padre Med Ctr / BOND, GERALD Schedule              CURRENT DATE
                                        04/11/12 - 04/12/12                             CURRENT TIME
=================================================================================================


04/11/12 Wednesday
   8:00a -  9:00a   *** BLOCKED              Rounds
  10:30a - 11:15a   ANDREWS, ANDY            LEFT HIP PAIN               (209) 746-9211
  12:00p -  1:00p   *** BLOCKED              Lunch
   1:00p -  1:45p   FISHER, ELOISE           INGUINAL HERNIA REPAIR      (209) 555-6111
   4:15p -  6:00p   *** BLOCKED              Unavailable

04/12/12 Thursday
   8:00a -  9:00a   *** BLOCKED              Unavailable
  10:30a - 11:15a   FLANNERY, SANDRA         RIGHT SHOULDER              (209) 555-8676
  11:15a - 11:45a   GROSS, BRIANNA           HUMERUS FRACTURE RECK       (209) 555-6116
  12:00p -  1:00p   *** BLOCKED              Lunch
   1:00p -  3:00p   GREGGORY, TERRY EMILY    L4/L5 LAMINECTOMY           (209) 555-6893
   3:00p -  4:30p   SMITH, CAROL             MICRODISCECTOMY             (209) 555-5286
   4:15p -  6:00p   *** BLOCKED              Unavailable


*** END OF PRINT  CURRENT DATE   CURRENT TIME ***
```

Figure 1-39: Dr. Bond's weekly schedule, which you are not to save

```
============================================================================================
PAGE - 1                     South Padre Med Ctr / BOND, GERALD Scheduled Visits      CURRENT DATE
                                              04/11/12                                CURRENT TIME
============================================================================================

04/11/12 Wednesday
   8:00a *B*L*O*C*K*E*D***************  Rounds                *B*L*O*C*K*E*D***************
   8:15a *B*L*O*C*K*E*D***************  Rounds                *B*L*O*C*K*E*D***************
   8:30a *B*L*O*C*K*E*D***************  Rounds                *B*L*O*C*K*E*D***************
   8:45a *B*L*O*C*K*E*D***************  Rounds                *B*L*O*C*K*E*D***************
   9:00a
   9:15a
   9:30a
   9:45a
  10:00a
  10:15a
  10:30a ANDREWS, ANDY               LEFT HIP PAIN           Texas Health Corporation    (209) 746-9211
  10:45a ANDREWS, ANDY               LEFT HIP PAIN           Texas Health Corporation    (209) 746-9211
  11:00a ANDREWS, ANDY               LEFT HIP PAIN           Texas Health Corporation    (209) 746-9211
  11:15a
  11:30a
  11:45a
  12:00p *B*L*O*C*K*E*D***************  Lunch                 *B*L*O*C*K*E*D***************
  12:15p *B*L*O*C*K*E*D***************  Lunch                 *B*L*O*C*K*E*D***************
  12:30p *B*L*O*C*K*E*D***************  Lunch                 *B*L*O*C*K*E*D***************
  12:45p *B*L*O*C*K*E*D***************  Lunch                 *B*L*O*C*K*E*D***************
   1:00p FISHER, ELOISE              INGUINAL HERNIA REPAIR  Texas Health Corporation    (209) 555-6111
   1:15p FISHER, ELOISE              INGUINAL HERNIA REPAIR  Texas Health Corporation    (209) 555-6111
   1:30p FISHER, ELOISE              INGUINAL HERNIA REPAIR  Texas Health Corporation    (209) 555-6111
   2:00p
   2:15p
   2:30p
   2:45p
   3:00p
   3:15p
   3:30p
   3:45p
   4:00p
   4:15p *B*L*O*C*K*E*D***************  Unavailable           *B*L*O*C*K*E*D***************
   4:30p *B*L*O*C*K*E*D***************  Unavailable           *B*L*O*C*K*E*D***************
   4:45p *B*L*O*C*K*E*D***************  Unavailable           *B*L*O*C*K*E*D***************
   5:00p *B*L*O*C*K*E*D***************  Unavailable           *B*L*O*C*K*E*D***************
   5:15p *B*L*O*C*K*E*D***************  Unavailable           *B*L*O*C*K*E*D***************
   5:30p *B*L*O*C*K*E*D***************  Unavailable           *B*L*O*C*K*E*D***************
   5:45p *B*L*O*C*K*E*D***************  Unavailable           *B*L*O*C*K*E*D***************

*** END OF PRINT  CURRENT DATE   CURRENT TIME ***
```

Figure 1-40: Dr. Bond's daily schedule for 04/11/12, which you are to save

```
PAGE - 1                    South Padre Med Ctr / BOND, GERALD Scheduled Visits            CURRENT DATE
                                              04/12/12                                      CURRENT TIME
```

04/12/12 Thursday
```
 8:00a *B*L*O*C*K*E*D***************  Unavailable          *B*L*O*C*K*E*D***************
 8:15a *B*L*O*C*K*E*D***************  Unavailable          *B*L*O*C*K*E*D***************
 8:30a *B*L*O*C*K*E*D***************  Unavailable          *B*L*O*C*K*E*D***************
 8:45a *B*L*O*C*K*E*D***************  Unavailable          *B*L*O*C*K*E*D***************
 9:00a
 9:15a
 9:30a
 9:45a
10:00a
10:15a
10:30a FLANNERY, SANDRA             RIGHT SHOULDER        Texas Medicare        (209) 555-8676
10:45a FLANNERY, SANDRA             RIGHT SHOULDER        Texas Medicare        (209) 555-8676
11:00a FLANNERY, SANDRA             RIGHT SHOULDER        Texas Medicare        (209) 555-8676
11:15a GROSS, BRIANNA               HUMERUS FRACTURE RECK  BC/BS of Texas       (209) 555-6116
11:30a GROSS, BRIANNA               HUMERUS FRACTURE RECK  BC/BS of Texas       (209) 555-6116
11:45a
12:00p *B*L*O*C*K*E*D***************  Lunch                *B*L*O*C*K*E*D***************
12:15p *B*L*O*C*K*E*D***************  Lunch                *B*L*O*C*K*E*D***************
12:30p *B*L*O*C*K*E*D***************  Lunch                *B*L*O*C*K*E*D***************
12:45p *B*L*O*C*K*E*D***************  Lunch                *B*L*O*C*K*E*D***************
 1:00p GREGGORY, TERRY EMILY        L4/L5 LAMINECTOMY                           (209) 555-6893
 1:15p GREGGORY, TERRY EMILY        L4/L5 LAMINECTOMY                           (209) 555-6893
 1:30p GREGGORY, TERRY EMILY        L4/L5 LAMINECTOMY                           (209) 555-6893
 1:45p GREGGORY, TERRY EMILY        L4/L5 LAMINECTOMY                           (209) 555-6893
 2:00p GREGGORY, TERRY EMILY        L4/L5 LAMINECTOMY                           (209) 555-6893
 2:15p GREGGORY, TERRY EMILY        L4/L5 LAMINECTOMY                           (209) 555-6893
 2:30p GREGGORY, TERRY EMILY        L4/L5 LAMINECTOMY                           (209) 555-6893
 2:45p GREGGORY, TERRY EMILY        L4/L5 LAMINECTOMY                           (209) 555-6893
 3:00p SMITH, CAROL                 MICRODISCECTOMY                             (209) 555-5286
 3:15p SMITH, CAROL                 MICRODISCECTOMY                             (209) 555-5286
 3:30p SMITH, CAROL                 MICRODISCECTOMY                             (209) 555-5286
 3:45p SMITH, CAROL                 MICRODISCECTOMY                             (209) 555-5286
 4:00p SMITH, CAROL                 MICRODISCECTOMY                             (209) 555-5286
 4:15p *B*L*O*C*K*E*D***************  Unavailable          *B*L*O*C*K*E*D***************
 4:15p SMITH, CAROL                 MICRODISCECTOMY                             (209) 555-5286
 4:30p *B*L*O*C*K*E*D***************  Unavailable          *B*L*O*C*K*E*D***************
 4:45p *B*L*O*C*K*E*D***************  Unavailable          *B*L*O*C*K*E*D***************
 5:00p *B*L*O*C*K*E*D***************  Unavailable          *B*L*O*C*K*E*D***************
 5:15p *B*L*O*C*K*E*D***************  Unavailable          *B*L*O*C*K*E*D***************
 5:30p *B*L*O*C*K*E*D***************  Unavailable          *B*L*O*C*K*E*D***************
 5:45p *B*L*O*C*K*E*D***************  Unavailable          *B*L*O*C*K*E*D***************
```

*** END OF PRINT CURRENT DATE   CURRENT TIME ***

Figure 1-41: Dr. Bond's daily schedule for 04/12/12, which you are to save

For Dr. Clark, save his schedule for 04/18/12.

- Save the document as LastName_YourFirstInitial_Task1.2Clark18

Task **1.3**

Entering Patient Data

Supplies Located on Evolve

- Gloria Hydorn's History and Physical Examination with Continuation form (Task 1.3 Hydorn Med Documents, contains 3 pages)

Dr. Adams performed a history and physical examination for Gloria Hydorn on Thursday, April 5, and you are now going to attach the documentation to the patient's record.

Obtain the medical document from the Evolve website and copy it into your Completed Work folder. Log in to the MedTrak software through the Evolve website and from the Main Menu, click **Scheduler**. Change the Location from South Padre Med Ctr to Gerald Bond and click **Submit Selection**. Click **Patients** to enter the area illustrated in Figure 1-42.

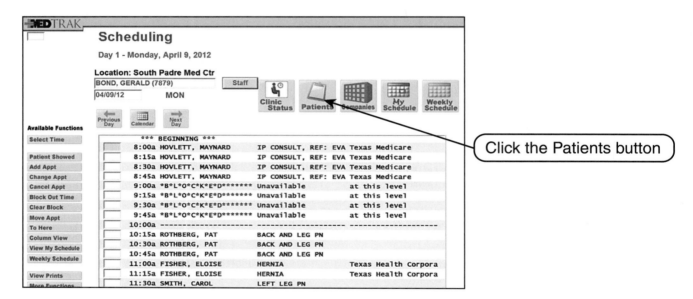

Figure 1-42: Accessing the patient database

In the Search field, type "Hydorn" (as illustrated in Figure 1-43) and then click **Search**.

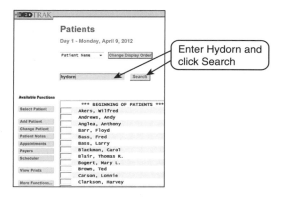

Figure 1-43: Searching for a patient in the patient database

When you click **Search**, Gloria Hydorn's name should appear at the top of the list. Type "DOC" in the block next to her name (as shown in Figure 1-44) and press **ENTER** on your keyboard.

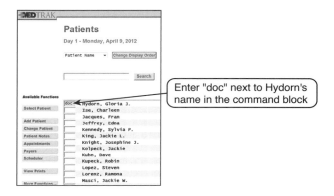

Figure 1-44: Attaching a document to a patient record

The next screen displays as shown in Figure 1-45. On the left side of the screen the Available Functions are View, Add, Delete, and Undelete. Click on the **Add** link.

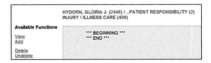

Figure 1-45: Adding documents to patient electronic medical records

Figure 1-46 illustrates the next screen, which is for adding a document to a patient record. Type "History and Physical" in the highlighted description area. Click the **Browse** button and locate your Completed Work folder, where you previously copied Gloria's medical documentation. Double-click this medical documentation in the folder and click the **Upload** button to upload the medical document to Gloria's EHR.

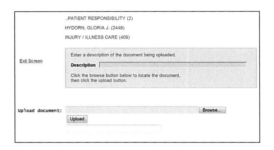

Figure 1-46: Description and uploading of external documents

You will know that your upload was successful when you see the screen shown in Figure 1-47.

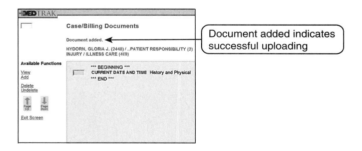

Figure 1-47: Document added indicates a successful uploading of a document to the EHR

Note that the Available Functions on the Case/Billing Documents screen, as illustrated in Figure 1-47, are again View, Add, Delete, and Undelete. Click **View** to display the document. Save this newly uploaded document to your Completed Work folder (Day 1, Task 1.3 subfolder) as LastName_YourFirstInitial_Task1.3Hydorn. Your next step is to delete the medical document you downloaded earlier for Gloria Hydorn from Evolve so that you only have one copy of the medical document for Gloria in your Completed Work folder. If your instructor asks for a copy of the document you uploaded into the EHR, this is the copy you will want to submit.

Exit the screen and return to the Main Menu.

Your final task for this day is to take a short ten-question quiz.

QUIZ

DAY 1

Using the MedTrak software, answer the following questions:

1. What patient is scheduled with Dr. Bond on Tuesday, April 10, at 10:30 a.m.?
   a. Gus Conrad
   b. Edwin Goldman
   c. Fran Jacques
   d. Lewis Rock

2. On Monday, April 9, Dr. Bond saw Eloise Fisher and asked you to schedule her for surgery. For what date and time did you schedule this surgery?
   a. 3 p.m. on 04/12/12
   b. 1 p.m. on 04/11/12
   c. 1 p.m. on 04/12/12
   d. 9 a.m. on 04/18/12

3. From a screen displaying a physician's schedule, what button would you click first to begin the process of printing the schedule?
   a. View Prints
   b. View My Schedule
   c. More Functions
   d. Select Time

4. You are looking at the Main Menu screen, and you click the Scheduling button. What is the default location displayed?
   a. South Padre Medical Center
   b. Dr. Bond's office
   c. Dr. Adams' office
   d. Dr. Harkness' office

5. There are two methods you can use to move the scheduler forward. One method is to click Calendar and move forward using the blue right and left arrows. Which is the other method?
   a. Type the date in the Location field
   b. Type the date in the Date field
   c. Click Calendar and click the left arrow only
   d. None of the methods above will move the date forward

6. From the Main Menu, if you click Clinic Status, how many exam and procedure rooms are listed under the four physicians' names?
   a. 10
   b. 9
   c. 8
   d. 6

7. From the Clinic Status view, to display the patient database, you would click which of the following?
   a. My Schedule
   b. Location
   c. More Functions
   d. Patients

8. According to Dr. Harkness' schedule for Wednesday, April 11, she is to see which patient at 4 p.m. in Consultation?
   a. Harriet Muir
   b. Jean Olson
   c. Jackie Masci
   d. Diana Morris

9. When you access the Scheduling function from the Main Menu and have the Location set on South Padre Medical Center, who is the first patient listed?
   a. Eloise Fisher
   b. David Oakland
   c. Pat Rothberg
   d. Maynard Hovlett

10. Who was the walk-in patient that you scheduled with Dr. Adams today?
    a. Emily Fisk
    b. Matt Fisher
    c. Kathy Forest
    d. Amanda Foster

To receive credit for your quiz, you **must** go to the Scheduler and in any command box (Figure 1-48) type "**QUIZ**" (upper, lower, or mixed case) and press **ENTER**.

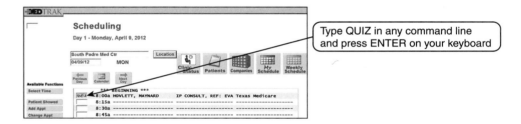

Figure 1-48: Closing out Day 1

The next screen you will see displays a box that says "I am done with the Quiz for Day 1." If you are done, click **Yes**. If you have not completed the quiz, click **No** and you will be returned to the scheduler.

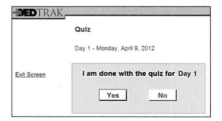

Figure 1-49: Dialog box for the completion of Day 1 quiz

After you have clicked the **Yes** button on the Day 1 Quiz dialog box, your screen will display **Day 2, Tuesday, April 10, 2012**, as shown in Figure 1-50.

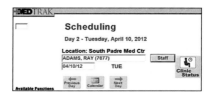

Figure 1-50: Successfully displaying Day 2, Tuesday, April 10, 2012

Congratulations! You have finished the first day of your internship, and you should feel very proud of yourself. It is not easy learning so many new things in such a short time, but you did it! Every day it will get a bit easier. Remember when you first rode a bike or drove a car? It was very difficult and at first you made a few mistakes. That is completely natural, and just as you conquered riding a bike or driving a car, these internship tasks will soon be second nature to you. Now go home, get some rest, and we will see you at the Center for Day 2.

Appointment Scheduling Guidelines

For billing purposes, a **new patient** is defined as one who has not seen the current physician or another physician of the same specialty at South Padre Medical Center within the past 3 years. An **established patient** is one who has seen any physician or another physician of the same specialty at the South Padre Medical Center within the past 3 years. An established patient's medical record is available and only needs to be updated. Because updating requires less time than does development of a new patient record, physicians get paid more for a new patient office visit than they do for an established patient visit. However, for purposes of the schedule, if the patient has been seen in the Center by any of the Center physicians, he or she is considered an established patient because a medical record is available for that patient.

It is your responsibility to schedule patient appointments and to ensure that the correct information is recorded on the appointment schedule. The physicians have developed a list of the length of time you should allow for the most common patient complaints. The scheduling guidelines on the next page (also presented in Appendix A and on the back inside cover of this Student Manual) should be used when you schedule new or established patients:

If a patient requires an appointment for a complaint not listed, use your judgment in making the appointment by basing the time on that required for the most similar complaint listed on the scheduling guidelines.

Appointment Scheduling Guidelines

15 MINUTES
- Allergies
- Bug bite
- Burn
- Cast recheck
- Conjunctivitis
- Cough
- Ear pain or infection
- Ear wash
- Elevated temperature
- Fall recheck
- Flu symptoms
- Pharyngitis
- Rash, hives
- Recheck flu
- Recheck Pap
- Sinus
- Sore throat
- URI
- UTI
- Wart treatment

30 MINUTES
- Abdominal pain
- Asthma
- Anxiety
- Back pain recheck
- Breast mass
- Bronchitis
- Cast change
- Chest congestion
- Chest pain
- Confusion
- Depression
- Diabetic new problem
- Diabetic recheck
- Dizziness
- Eye injury
- Foreign body removal (location)
- Headache
- Hernia
- Hip pain recheck
- Infection
- Ingrown toenail
- Laceration, head, arm, hand
- Leg pain recheck
- Lesion removal (1)
- Medication recheck
- Menstrual problems

- Muscle strain
- OB check
- Pap
- Postoperative visit
- Preop physical
- Shortness of breath (SOB)
- Sprain or suspected fracture
- STD
- Stiff neck
- Varicocele recheck

45 MINUTES
- Back pain
- Breast pain
- Dog bite
- Hip pain
- Knee pain
- Laceration, trunk, leg
- Leg pain
- Lump
- Neck pain
- Shoulder pain
- Varicose veins
- Postoperative complication or pain

60 MINUTES
- Establish physician
- Initial OB

PHYSICALS/PAPS
15 to 60 MINUTES
- Pap included for female patients (over age 18)
- Physicals (px) and preoperatives (preop) (schedule by age)

Under 18	15 minutes
18-40	30 minutes
41-65	45 minutes
Over 65	60 minutes

CONSULTATION
Request for an inpatient consultation: Prefer an hour but can schedule for 45 minutes. Note reason for consultation and requesting physician when placing inpatient consultation on schedule.

CARDIAC 1 HOUR
- New cardiac outpatient
- New inpatient consultation

SURGERY SCHEDULING
45 MINUTES
- Cholecystectomy, laparoscopic
- Fracture repair
- Hearing check
- Lesion removal (2 or more)
- Outpatient echocardiogram
- Proctosigmoidoscopy (procto)
- Hernia repair

60 MINUTES
- Appendectomy, laparoscopic
- Breast biopsy
- Cardiac catheterization
- Hernia repair with graft
- Initial (new) OB visit
- Kidney biopsy
- Liver biopsy
- Lymph biopsy
- Lymphadenectomy
- Mastectomy
- Needle biopsy
- New surgical patient
- Pacemaker
- Septoplasty
- Surgical echocardiogram

90 MINUTES
- Decompression, arthroscopic, such as, shoulder
- Discectomy
- GI bypass, laparoscopic
- Microdiscectomy

120 MINUTES
- Hip, closed reduction and screw placement
- Knee, total arthroplasty
- Meniscectomy
- Laminectomy, foraminotomies, facetectomies
- Tendon, open repair

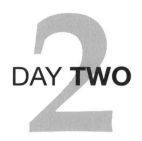

DAY **TWO**

Tuesday, April 10, 2012

TASK **2.1**	Printing Daily Schedules
TASK **2.2**	Scheduling Consultations and Hospital Admissions
TASK **2.3**	Locating Patient Data
TASK **2.4**	Scheduling Surgeries and Return Appointments

TASK **2.1**

PRINTING DAILY SCHEDULES

 ## *Requirements*

- Access to MedTrak software

Good morning! Glad to see you for Day 2 of your internship. Gladys has asked that you print the schedules for both Dr. Bond and Dr. Adams for today. Yesterday, you learned how to print a daily schedule, so if you have questions on how to do the task, refer to the directions previously provided. Save a copy of Dr. Bond's and Dr. Adams' schedules for Tuesday, April 10, 2012, in your Completed Work folder as follows:

- LastName_YourFirstInitial_Task2.1Bond
- LastName_YourFirstInitial_Task2.1Adams

Task 2.2

SCHEDULING CONSULTATIONS AND HOSPITAL ADMISSIONS

Dr. Bond called the office and informed Gladys that he has been at the hospital since early this morning providing a consultation for Eugena Dore, a patient Dr. Adams admitted last night. Dr. Bond has requested that we schedule Eugena for left hip fracture repair surgery this afternoon at 3:45 p.m. Your first step is to remove the "Unavailable" blocking from 8-9 a.m. from Dr. Bond's schedule and add an appointment for a consultation for Eugena, as illustrated in Figure 2-1. (Remember to click the **Location** button to change to Dr. Bond.) Do not use the **Block Out Time** button to add the consultation; rather, use the **Add Appt** button, search for Dore, select the patient, and indicate a 60-minute appointment for an Inpatient Consultation.

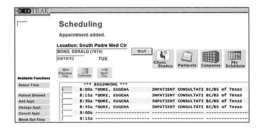

Figure 2-1: Eugena Dore added to the schedule as Inpatient Consultation

Dr. Bond has scheduled Eugena Dore for surgery at 3:45 p.m. today after his appointment with Edward Goldman. Although this is not Dr. Bond's usual surgery day, he has decided to perform Eugena's surgery today. First, remove any blocking on Dr. Bond's schedule for this afternoon. Block out 15 minutes of travel time after the Goldman appointment to allow Dr. Bond time to travel to the hospital. Eugena will have a closed reduction and screw placement of the left hip for fracture repair, which you can indicate on the appointment as the reason (L Hip Fx Repair). Refer to the appointment scheduling guidelines for the length of time to schedule for this procedure. If there is any time left after Eugena's surgery, block the remaining time as "Unavailable."

Dr. Bond has to return to the hospital after his center appointment with Lewis Rock later today to provide a consultation for Dr. Bethos' patient, Thomas J. Blair. Gladys has registered the patient in the patient database and now wants you to record this appointment on Dr. Bond's schedule. Schedule travel from 11:15-11:30 with the consultation to follow. The patient is going to be seen in the outpatient (OP) setting at the hospital. Dr. Bond will use his lunchtime to finish the consultation, so Gladys directs you to schedule 60 minutes for the Outpatient Consultation beginning at 11:30 a.m., even though the appointment will overlap with Dr. Bond's scheduled lunch break. Record the reason as "Outpatient Consultation."

After you have completed scheduling Eugena, save a copy of Dr. Bond's schedule for Tuesday, April 10, 2012, in your Completed Work folder as LastName_YourFirstInitial_Task2.2Bond.

Last night, Dr. Adams admitted Eugena into the hospital. He brought a note to the office early this morning indicating that we are to place her on the schedule today from 8-9 a.m. to ensure the service is on the schedule. Remove the blocking from 8-9 a.m. and replace it with a 1-hour appointment for Eugena Dore with the reason as "Hospital Admit." Save a copy of Dr. Adams' new schedule for today in your Completed Work folder as LastName_YourFirstInitial_Task2.2Adams.

Gladys wants to know when Dave Kuhn has been scheduled for an appointment and for surgery. She requests that you access the patient's EHR and inform her of the time and date of this previously scheduled appointment and surgery. To do this, click **Patient Registration**, and do a search for Kuhn. When Dave Kuhn's name is displayed on the top of the patient search, click in the command box next to his name and click the **Appointments** button on the left. Keep this screen open while you complete the following exercise.

Exercise 2-1

Using the information that displayed after you clicked Appointments above, answer questions 1 and 2:

1. The time of Dave's surgery is on _____ at _____ p.m.

2. Dave's appointment is on _____ at _____ p.m. with Dr. _____.

Using the same process to locate Jasper Hunt's record, answer questions 3 and 4:

3. Jasper is schedule for an appointment on _____ at _____ with Dr. _____.

4. Nellie Groff has an appointment on _____ at _____ a.m. with Dr. _____.

 Gladys wants you to download an inpatient orthopedic consultation document from the Evolve website for a consultation that Dr. Bond provided for Maynard Hovlett, a patient of Dr. Evans. The date of the consultation was yesterday, 04/09/12. Use the directions for attaching a document that you learned on Day 1 when you attached a document to Gloria Hydorn's EHR. Remember to save a copy of the report to your Completed Work folder as LastName_YourFirstInitial_Task2.2Hovlett.

DAY TWO   TASK 2.2

Task 2.3

LOCATING PATIENT DATA

Gladys wants to show you how easy it is to locate patient information located in the patient database using the MedTrak software. From the Main Menu, click the **Patient Registration** button. In the highlighted Search box on the Patients screen, type "Hoverson" and click the **Search** button at the end of the box. You have searched and located patients using this search feature before, so this is not new; however, you are now going to learn about a new way to access patient information. In the Command box next to Adam G. Hoverson's name, key in "Appt" and click **ENTER** on your keyboard. The screen will next display an appointment Adam had at the Center yesterday, 04/09/12, with Dr. Adams, as illustrated in Figure 2-2.

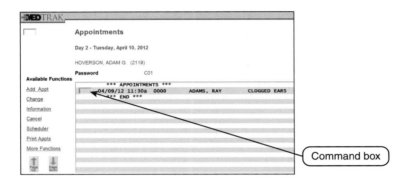

Figure 2-2: Appointment screen for Adam G. Hoverson

Place your cursor in the command box next to Adam's name and click **Information** on the left side of the screen. The Contact Information screen will display patient, insurance, and appointment information, as illustrated in Figure 2-3.

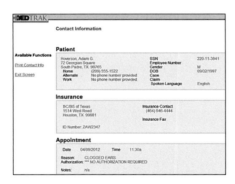

Figure 2-3: Contact Information screen for Adam G. Hoverson

Click the **Print Contact Info** link on the left side of the screen. Although no prompt appears, a copy of the contact information has been sent to the printer. Let's locate this document. Click **Exit Screen** to return to the Appointments screen. Click the **Exit Screen** command again; this takes you to the Patients screen. Now click **View Prints** on the left side of the screen, and you will see an Appointment Information Report ready to print. Open the document and then save a copy in your Completed Work folder as LastName_YourFirstInitial_Task2.3Hoverson.

Exercise 2-2

Use the same search feature you just learned about to locate patient Contact Information and answer the following questions.

1. According to the Contact Information for Eloise Fisher, she has Texas Health Corporation insurance. What is the ID number of that company? _____

2. Pat Rothberg had an appointment on 04/09/12. What was the reason for this appointment? _____

3. Sylvia P. Kennedy had an appointment with Dr. Adams on 04/09/12. At what time was the appointment? _____

4. Jackie W. Masci was referred to Dr. Clark by Dr. Adams. What was the reason for this referral? _____

Task **2.4**

SCHEDULING SURGERIES AND RETURN APPOINTMENTS

This day has gone by very quickly, with so many things to do and learn. Gladys has another project that she would like you to complete. It is one that you should be familiar with now that you have scheduled several surgeries.

Access Dr. Bond's schedule to place a patient on his surgery schedule. The patient is Edward A. Goldman, who was seen in the office today at 2:30 p.m. Dr. Bond wants the patient placed on his 04/19/12 surgery schedule at 1 p.m. for a meniscectomy. The surgery is scheduled to start at 1 p.m. When you are finished, save a copy of Dr. Bond's 04/19/12 schedule in your Completed Work folder as LastName_YourFirstInitial_Task2.4Bond.

Next, you need to schedule a return appointment for Jasper Hunt, who saw Dr. Adams today. Jasper would like his return appointment to be on 04/19/12. Gladys instructs you to schedule a 30-minute appointment at 10 a.m. for a strain recheck. Save a copy of Dr. Adams schedule for 04/19/12 in your Completed Work folder as LastName_YourFirstInitial_Task2.4Adams.

Your final task before you are finished for this day is to take a short ten-question quiz.

Quiz

DAY 2

Using the MedTrak software, answer the following questions:

1. What patient is scheduled with Dr. Bond on Tuesday, April 10, at 10:30 a.m.?
   a. Brianna Gross
   b. Jasper Hunt
   c. Fran Jacques
   d. Lewis Rock

2. On Tuesday, April 10, Dr. Bond saw Edward A. Goldman and asked you to schedule him for surgery. What was the date and time you scheduled for this patient?
   a. 1 p.m. on 04/19/12
   b. 1 p.m. on 04/11/12
   c. 1 p.m. on 04/12/12
   d. 9 a.m. on 04/18/12

3. From a screen displaying a physician's schedule, what button would you click first to begin the process of printing the schedule?
   a. Add Appt
   b. Change Appt
   c. More Functions
   d. Patient Showed

4. From the Main Menu screen, what button do you click to access the screen that displays the exam rooms?
   a. Patient Registration
   b. Scheduler
   c. Administration
   d. Clinic Status

5. From the Main Menu, when you click the Patient Registration button and do a search for Dennis Dross, what is his birthdate?
   a. 02/20/1945
   b. 03/27/1955
   c. 08/04/1977
   d. 11/13/1943

6. Who is the first person on Dr. Harkness' schedule for 04/11/12?
   a. Steven Lopez
   b. George Sorenson
   c. Bertha Wilson
   d. Harvey Clarkson

7. From the Main Menu, when you click the Scheduler button, which patient's name appears twice at 8 a.m.?
   a. Tom Syefer
   b. Edward Goldman
   c. Peter Silverman
   d. Eugena Dore

8. What is the name of the patient who is scheduled with Dr. Clark for a gastric bypass at 9 a.m. on 04/12/12?
   a. Harriet Muir
   b. Jean Olson
   c. Jackie Masci
   d. Diana Morris

9. What is on Dr. Adams' schedule for tomorrow, Wednesday, April 11, at 8 a.m.?
   a. Medical School
   b. Rounds
   c. Board meeting
   d. Unavailable

10. You uploaded a document and attached it to Maynard Hovlett's EHR. According to that document, the radiographs were performed on which body part?
    a. Back
    b. Hand
    c. Hip
    d. Knee

It's time to receive credit for your quiz! Remember that you **must** go to the Scheduler, type "**QUIZ**" in any command line, and press **ENTER**. The next screen you will see displays a box that says "I am done with the Quiz for Day 2." If you are done, click **Yes**. If you have not completed the quiz, click No and you will be returned to the Scheduler. After you have clicked the **Yes** button on the Day 2 Quiz dialog box, your screen will display **Day 2 completed, Day 3 (April 11, 2012) charts loaded**.

Another day of your internship has been successfully completed! You are making great progress and learning a great deal about working in the electronic health record environment. We look forward to seeing you again tomorrow. You worked really hard today and should feel great about your accomplishments!

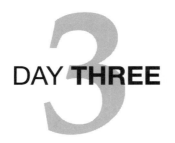

DAY THREE

Wednesday, April 11, 2012

TASK **3.1**   Scheduling Appointments and Surgery

TASK **3.2**   Records Management

TASK **3.3**   Sorting Mail

TASK **3.4**   Petty Cash

TASK **3.1**

SCHEDULING APPOINTMENTS AND SURGERY

 Requirements

- Access to MedTrak software

This is the start of Day 3 of your internship and there are many interesting things to learn today. Today, Gladys has asked that you schedule the following patients on the physicians' schedules:

- Dr. Bond called Gladys and asked that his morning schedule be revised to accommodate a patient. The patient, Lori Whittaker, is an inpatient whose attending physician, Dr. Bethos, has requested a consultation. Enter Lori on Dr. Bond's schedule for today from 8-9 a.m. as a "Consult, Bethos," which will be a 60-minute service. You cannot book over a blocked time, so first clear the blocking from 8-9 and then using the **Add Appt** button, schedule the patient's appointment according to Dr. Bond's instructions.

- Dr. Bond also has scheduled Lori for surgery this afternoon at 2 p.m. for a closed reduction of a hip fracture with placement of screws. You will be copying all the physicians' schedules at the end of the day, so you do not need to copy Dr. Bond's schedule at this time.

- Dr. Harkness has asked Gladys to enter a cardiology consultation for Floyd Barr, an inpatient, to start at 8 a.m. today. Her time is blocked for rounds, but she has asked that the Barr consultation, requested by Dr. Adams, be recorded on her schedule and the rounds removed.

- Dr. Harkness has scheduled Floyd for a cardiac catheterization at 11 a.m. this morning and requests that the appointment be recorded on her schedule.

- Dr. Bond has seen Andy Andrews this morning and wants the patient scheduled for a left hip decompression on Friday, 04/20/12, at 1 p.m. Dr. Bond has decided to do this surgery even though it is not usually on his surgical schedule. Dr. Bond has requested that his schedule be unblocked from 1-6 p.m. that day to allow for other procedures to be scheduled. After you have unblocked his Friday schedule from 1-6 p.m. and added the appointment for Andy Andrews, reblock the remaining time as "Surgery" so that others will know that other surgical procedures may be added to the schedule during the remaining time on Friday.

- Gus Conrad is a walk-in patient at 10:30 a.m. He has stomach pain with pressure and vomiting and wants to see a physician. Gladys enters the patient into the database and asks that you schedule him with Dr. Adams at 10:45 a.m.

DAY THREE   TASK 3.1

- Jason Eskew is also a walk-in at 11:05 a.m. and Gladys has entered his information in the patient database. She asks that you schedule Jason with Dr. Bond at 11:15 a.m. today for the reason of "Arm/Shoulder Pain" for 45 minutes.

- Dr. Bond has requested that the time from 4-4:15 p.m. today be blocked as "Unavailable" because he has some hospital rounds he wants to attend to after his last scheduled surgery.

- Dr. Harkness asks you to schedule Harriet Muir for insertion of a pacemaker on Thursday, April 12, 2012, at noon. The patient is a referral from Dr. Evans, so record the reason as "Pacemaker, Ref Evans."

Gladys asks you to copy the six daily schedules to your Completed Work folder for Day 3, Task 3.1, as follows:

- Dr. Bond's schedule for 04/11/12 as LastName_YourFirstInitial_Task3.1Bond11 and his 04/20/12 schedule as LastName_YourFirstInitial_Task3.1Bond20

- Dr. Adams' schedule for 04/11/12 as LastName_YourFirstInitial_Task3.1Adams

- Dr. Harkness' schedule for 04/11/12 as LastName_YourFirstInitial_Task3.1Harkness11 and her schedule for 04/12/12 as LastName_YourFirstInitial_Task3.1Harkness12

- Dr. Clark's schedule for 04/11/12 as LastName_YourFirstInitial_Task3.1Clark (there were no changes on this schedule today)

Time now to move on from scheduling to a new task that Gladys thinks you will enjoy.

Task **3.2**

RECORDS MANAGEMENT

Last night, Dr. Adams was called to the hospital to care for patient Floyd Barr, who was presented to the emergency department with chest and back pain. Dr. Sutton, an emergency department physician provided the initial ED care for the patient and ordered a chest x-ray. Dr. Sutton then notified Dr. Adams because Dr. Adams is Floyd's primary care physician. Dr. Adams subsequently admitted Floyd to the hospital. Dr. Adams requested a consultation by Dr. Harkness. You are to attach these three documents to Floyd Barr's EHR and name the documents you attach as follows:

- Emergency Department
- Radiology Report
- Admission

You have attached documents to medical records in previous tasks; therefore, Gladys asks you to attach documents again, without further direction. When you have successfully attached the documents, your screen will appear as in Figure 3-1.

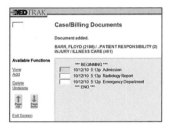

Figure 3-1: Attaching medical documents to Floyd Barr's EHR

Dr. Bond provided an orthopedic consultation for an outpatient of Dr. Bethos on Tuesday, 04/10/12. Gladys directs you to attach the document to the patient's EHR. The patient was Thomas J. Blair.

Gladys also wants you to attach medical documentation to Eugena Dore's EHR. Eugena was brought by ambulance to the emergency department. Dr. Adams admitted the patient and requested an orthopedic consultation with Dr. Bond, who consulted and later that day performed a closed reduction procedure. Attach these four documents to Eugena's EHR:

- Emergency Department
- Initial Hospital Care
- Orthopedic Consultation
- Operative Report

Exercise 3-1

Accessing the reports you just attached to the patient's EHR, answer these questions:

1. According to Floyd Barr's admission document, skin grafting is listed as a past surgery of the _____ leg.

2. According to Floyd Barr's radiology report, the 04/10/12 examination was compared with a prior examination dated _____ .

3. According to Eugena Dore's emergency department report, the chief complaint was pain in the _____ .

4. According to Eugena Dore's operative report, the estimated blood loss was _____ cc.

Task **3.3**

SORTING MAIL

Supplies Located on Evolve

- Mail Sorting form (Figure 3-2)
- Incoming Mail form dated April 11 (Figure 3-3)

Gladys has given you instructions to sort the incoming mail by person and department. You will get all of the mail from the Incoming Mail form (see Figure 3-3). You will sort the mail by physician, insurance, accounts receivable, human resources, waiting room, and Gladys. You will indicate the mail received under the appropriate heading (see Figure 3-2)—for example, Dr. Bond receives pieces of mail 1 and 17.

MAIL SORTING

Dr. Bond
1, 17

Dr. Harkness

Dr. Adams

Dr. Clark

Gladys

Accounts receivable

Insurance

Human Resources

Waiting Room

Figure 3-2: Incoming Mail sorting form for Wednesday, April 11

```
┌─────────────────────────────────────────────────────────────────┐
│                    INCOMING MAIL FORM                             │
│                    WEDNESDAY, APRIL 11                             │
│                                                                   │
│    1.  Letter to Dr. Bond from Dr. Andrews                        │
│    2.  BC/BS of TX (payments)                                     │
│    3.  Good Housekeeping magazine (Dr. Harkness's office)         │
│    4.  Completed job applications from Job Service of TX          │
│    5.  Letter from the Medicare Appeals Division                  │
│    6.  Pathology results State of Texas Pathology, Attn: Dr. Adams│
│    7.  Texas Health (payments)                                    │
│    8.  People Magazine (Dr. Adams' office)                        │
│    9.  X-ray pouches for Dr. Clark                                │
│   10.  Blank IRS/W-4 forms                                        │
│   11.  Envelope containing CMS-1500 forms, attn: Kerri Marshall   │
│   12.  Personal marked letter to Dr. Harkness                     │
│   13.  3 boxes of check blanks/South Padre Medical Center         │
│   14.  South Padre Living (2 copies, magazine)                    │
│   15.  1 box from South Padre Printing Company containing letterhead stationery │
│   16.  BC/BS of TX Appeals Division                               │
│   17.  Gold Prospector magazine (Dr. Gerald Bond)                 │
│   18.  4 boxes of business cards, one for each Dr. in the clinic  │
│   19.  Request for surgical consultation for Dr. Clark            │
│   20.  Medicare (reimbursement)                                   │
└─────────────────────────────────────────────────────────────────┘
```

Figure 3-3: Incoming Mail form for Wednesday, April 11

Gladys wants you to read the Center's guidelines before you complete the mail sorting task.

Guidelines on Sorting Incoming Mail

The U.S. Postal Service delivers the mail each day between 9 and 10 a.m. The front desk receptionist receives the mail and does the initial sorting. The mail should be sorted and handled as follows:

1. **Patients' laboratory or pathology results**

   - Scan the results and write "rec'd" and the date received (i.e., 04/11/12) in the upper right-hand corner of each report, as illustrated in Figure 3-4. Results that are positive are of the greatest priority.

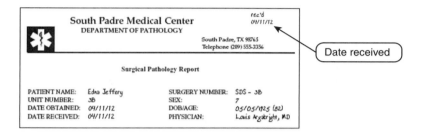

Figure 3-4: Date received

   - Positive results are to be placed on the top of the physician's incoming mail stack for immediate physician attention. If the physician is out of the office for more than a day, give the results to the physician's nurse.
   - Negative results are to be put in a file folder and placed in the physician's mail stack to be reviewed and initialed before the reports are uploaded to the EHR.

DAY THREE TASK 3.3

2. **Mail marked "Personal" or "Confidential"**

- These items are not to be opened by you, but instead placed on the mail stack as they were received. Write "rec'd" and the date received on the front of the envelope in the lower left-hand corner, as illustrated in Figure 3-5.

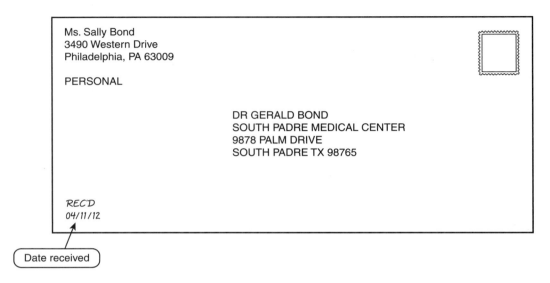

Ms. Sally Bond
3490 Western Drive
Philadelphia, PA 63009

PERSONAL

DR GERALD BOND
SOUTH PADRE MEDICAL CENTER
9878 PALM DRIVE
SOUTH PADRE TX 98765

REC'D
04/11/12

Date received

Figure 3-5: Personal or confidential mail

3. **Important letters, memos, documents**

- Open the mail and date-stamp each item.
- Review each item to ensure that it cannot be handled by another Center employee. When you are a new employee, you are to review these mail items with your supervisor/trainer until you are familiar with the office team and each employee's duties.

4. **Payments from patients or insurance companies**

- Sort the payments into two stacks—one for patient payments and the other for insurance company payments.
- Payments are to be delivered to accounts receivable.
- Place the envelope in which the payment was received behind each check or cash payment. Secure together the envelope, payment, and any correspondence that accompanied the payment with a paper clip. This step, which is especially important for cash payments, will ensure that all payments are credited to the correct accounts.

5. **Financial documents**

- Center bank statements, invoices, payroll forms, and state and federal tax information are to be dated and grouped together.

6. **Medical newsletters, journals, periodicals**

   - These medical materials are to be delivered to the physician to whom they are addressed and are never to be placed in the patient waiting room.

7. **Reception room magazines and newspapers**

   - People, Good Housekeeping, and other general reading magazines are to be placed in the waiting room.
   - Some physicians have personal magazine subscriptions sent to the office. These personal magazines are to be delivered to the physician, not placed in the waiting room. Dr. Bond's personal subscriptions are RV World and Gold Prospector magazines. Dr. Adams subscribes to Money Monthly and Downhill Ski.

8. **Advertisements**

   - Deliver these to Gladys.

9. **Other**

   - Stationery, business cards, check blanks, and other items from a printer are to be delivered to Gladys, who will review and approve the items for distribution or storage.

Delivery Service Items

A variety of services deliver packages and letters to the Center each day (e.g., Federal Express, United Parcel Service, private delivery services). The times for these deliveries vary; however, deliveries are usually made before 4 p.m. each day. When a service delivers an item, you are to follow the same procedures as outlined for the U.S. mail service. Many of the supplies for the Center arrive by delivery service, and when a department item is received, you should notify the department to whom the package is addressed immediately by telephone. Write the department name on the top of the item in order to facilitate pickup by department personnel. Set these items under the reception counter for pickup by the receiving department's personnel.

Once you have completed this part of Task 3.3, place the Mail Sorting form in your Completed Work folder.

Exercise 3-2

Using the Mail Sorting document you just completed, answer the following questions:

1. The letter from the Medicare Appeals Division was sorted to go to which department? _____

2. The x-ray pouches were for which physician? _____

3. Who received the copy of Gold Prospector magazine? _____

4. The Medicare reimbursements were sorted to go where? _____

DAY THREE TASK 3.3

Task **3.4**

PETTY CASH

 Supplies Located on Evolve

- Petty Cash Journal
- Center check, #999

Gladys has asked you to write a check for $100 to be used to set up a petty cash fund for the office. The check is to be written paid to the order of "First National Bank-Cash" and recorded on the check register. The address of the bank is to be listed on lines 2 and 3 under the payee on the sample check, in the area to the right of "TO THE ORDER OF," as illustrated in Figure 3-6. When you have the check prepared, begin the petty cash journal that Gladys drafted by entering the beginning balance of $100 at the top right-hand corner of the journal. The journal will be used to keep track of how the petty cash funds are spent.

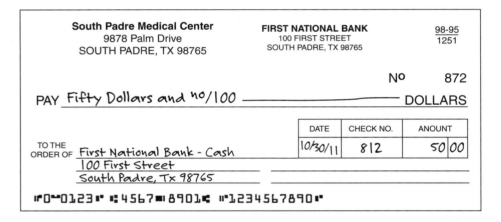

Figure 3-6: Sample check

Your only task left before you are finished for the day is to take the following short ten-question quiz.

Quiz

DAY 3

Using the MedTrak software, answer the following questions:

1. What patient is scheduled with Dr. Bond on Wednesday, April 11, at 10:30 a.m.?
   a. Andy Andrews
   b. Jasper Hunt
   c. Fran Jacques
   d. Sandra Flannery

2. On Wednesday, April 11, Dr. Harkness saw Floyd Barr and asked you to schedule him for a cardiac catheterization. What was the date and time you scheduled for Mr. Barr?
   a. 11 a.m. on 04/12/12
   b. 11 a.m. on 04/11/12
   c. 1 p.m. on 04/12/12
   d. 9 a.m. on 04/18/12

3. According to the admission report that you uploaded to Floyd Barr's EHR, the patient had cataract surgery of what?
   a. The right eye
   b. The left eye
   c. Both eyes
   d. Neither eye

4. According to the radiology report that you uploaded to Floyd Barr's EHR, who was the radiologist who prepared the report?
   a. Paul Sutton, MD
   b. Bert Bethos, MD
   c. Grey Lonewolf, MD
   d. Morton Monson, MD

5. According to the ED report that you uploaded to Floyd Barr's EHR, who was the ED physician?
   a. Paul Sutton, MD
   b. Bert Bethos, MD
   c. Grey Lonewolf, MD
   d. Morton Monson, MD

6. According to the orthopedic consultation report you uploaded for Eugena Dore, what was the admitting diagnosis?
   a. Intertrochanteric fracture of left hip
   b. Intertrochanteric fracture of right hip
   c. Intertrochanteric fractures of right and left hip
   d. Intertrochanteric fracture, site unspecified

7. According to the initial hospital care report you uploaded for Eugena Dore, which of the following is not listed in the Medications section of the report?
   a. Lisinopril, 20 mg a day
   b. Hydrochlorothiazide, 12.5 mg a day
   c. Alendronate, 90 mg every Sunday
   d. Vitamin D

8. According to the procedure on sorting the mail that arrives at the Center, what are you directed to do with personal mail addressed to a physician?
    a. Open it promptly
    b. Deliver it to your supervisor
    c. Take it immediately to the physician to whom it is addressed
    d. Mark it as received, record the date it was received, and place it on the mail stack unopened

9. Which of the following correctly describes the initial sorting of payments received from patient and insurance companies?
    a. One stack for patient payments and one stack for insurance company payments delivered to accounts receivable
    b. Payments not sorted, but delivered in one stack to accounts receivable
    c. One stack for both patient and insurance company payments delivered to Gladys
    d. One stack for patient payments and one stack for insurance company payments delivered to Gladys

10. What was the amount for which you wrote a check and initiated the Petty Cash Fund?
    a. $1,000
    b. $100
    c. $250
    d. $10

It's time to receive credit for your quiz! Remember that you **must** go to the Scheduler, type "**QUIZ**" in any command line, and press **ENTER**. The next screen you will see displays a box that says "I am done with the Quiz for Day 3." If you are done, click **Yes**. If you have not completed the quiz, click **No** and you will be returned to the Scheduler. After you have clicked the **Yes** button on the Day 3 Quiz dialog box, your screen will display **Day 3 completed, Day 4 (April 12, 2012) charts loaded**.

It is already Thursday tomorrow, and you are very close to being finished with your first week of internship. What an accomplishment!

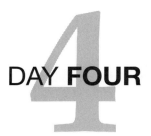

DAY **FOUR**

Thursday, April 12, 2012

TASK **4.1**	Accounts Receivable and Invoices
TASK **4.2**	Scheduling Proofing and Revisions
TASK **4.3**	Attaching Documents
TASK **4.4**	Internet Research

TASK **4.1**

ACCOUNTS RECEIVABLE AND INVOICES

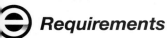 *Requirements*

- Access to MedTrak software

This is the start of Day 4 of your internship, and today you are going to learn some new functions using the MedTrak system. The first task will be billing, so let's get started. From the Main Menu, click the **Billing** button, as displayed in Figure 4-1.

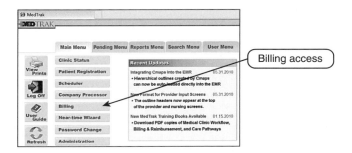

Figure 4-1: Billing access

The screen you access is shown in Figure 4-2. Click the **Unbilled Dashboard**, which takes you to the Unbilled Charges screen.

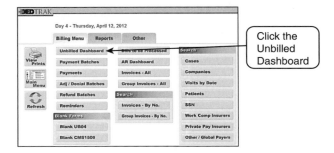

Figure 4-2: The Billing Menu

The Unbilled Charges screen appears in Figure 4-3. In the "Completed visits" section of the screen, under the heading "Charges available for review," locate the blue linked number directly under Patient. Click on that blue linked number.

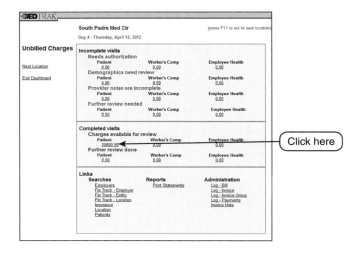

Figure 4-3: Unbilled Charges screen

You will be presented with the Unbilled Charges: Patient, Ready to Post screen, as shown in Figure 4-4. Place your cursor in the command block next to COMM INS; when that block is highlighted, click the **Select Class** button on the left side of the screen.

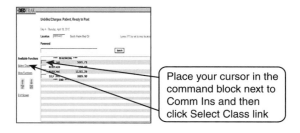

Figure 4-4: Selecting Commercial Insurance

The next screen displays the Unbilled Charges: Patient, COMM INS. By default, the display is by date of service, as illustrated in Figure 4-5. Click the **View** button.

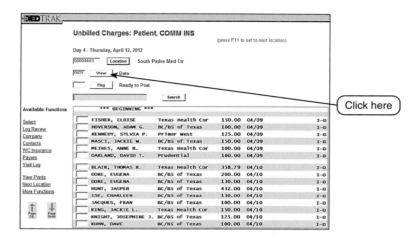

Figure 4-5: Patients in the Unbilled Charges area

When you click **View**, the screen displays the Unbilled Charges/View screen, as shown in Figure 4-6. Check the command box next to "PATT-Patient." When that block is checked and highlighted, click the **Submit Selection** button on the left of the screen.

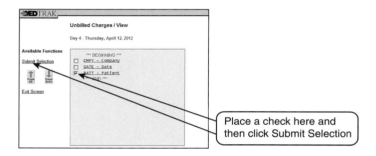

Figure 4-6: Unbilled Charges/View

Once you select the patient view, the Unbilled Charges: Patient, COMM INS screen will again appear, but this time the charges are listed in alphabetic order by patient, as illustrated in Figure 4-7. Place your cursor in the command box next to the name "Andrews, Andy" and click the **Select** link on the left side of the screen.

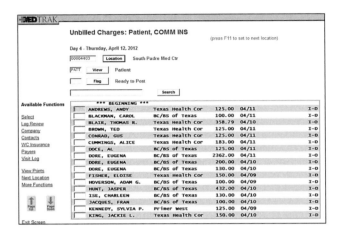

Figure 4-7: Patients in the Unbilled Charges area in order by patient name

When you have clicked the **Select** button, you will see the detailed Visit Information screen, as shown in Figure 4-8. With the command box highlighted next to "Level of Service," click the **Show Charges** link on the left side of the screen to display the charges for the selected service.

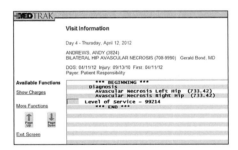

Figure 4-8: Visit Information screen

With your computer displaying the details of the visit charges, place your cursor in the command box next to "ofc visit ..." on the first line and click the **Post Charges** link on the left side of the screen, as illustrated in Figure 4-9.

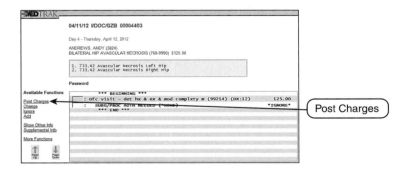

Figure 4-9: Display of details of the visit charges

When you click the **Post Charges** link, the charges are posted and you are automatically returned to the Unbilled Charges: Patient, Ready to Post screen, where you can select another patient with charges to post, such as Carol Blackman. Gladys has reviewed all the unbilled charges and has given you permission to approve them all. Post all the Unbilled Charges now. When you have posted all the unbilled charges, there will be no patient names displayed in the Unbilled Charges area, which means that you posted all the charges for patients with commercial insurance, but you still have to post charges for Medicaid, Medicare, and Self-Pay. To continue to post the other charges, click **Exit Screen** until you are returned to the Unbilled Charges: Patient, Ready to Post screen, as shown in Figure 4-10.

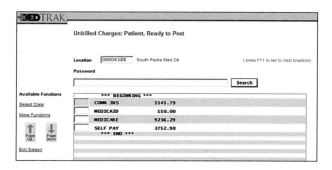

Figure 4-10: Returning to the Unbilled Charges screen

Once you have returned to the Unbilled Charges screen, place your cursor in the Medicaid command box and click the **Select Class** link on the left side of the screen. Then approve all the charges on that Unbilled Charges screen for Medicaid as you did for the commercial insurance charges. When you have posted all the charges for Medicaid, move to the Medicare and Self-Pay charges. Approve charges until you have posted all the charges on the Unbilled Charges screen. When you have posted all charges, exit the screen and navigate back to the Billing Menu. From the Billing Menu, select **Bills to be Processed**, as illustrated in Figure 4-11.

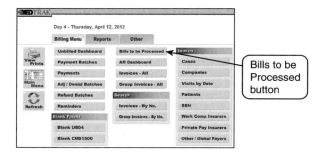

Figure 4-11: Billing Menu, Bills to be Processed

The next screen will be as illustrated in Figure 4-12. Note that there are three sections on the main part of the screen: "Printed," "Electronically," and "Total all bills," along with a "Number" column and an "Amount" column. The "Total all bills" section shows the total number of bills to be processed and the amount of the total bills. In the "Printed" section, place your cursor in the "Patient - Invoices" command box (indicated by the arrow in Figure 4-12) and click the **View Bills** link on the left side of the screen.

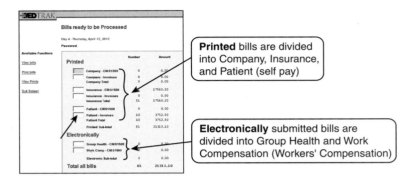

Figure 4-12: Bills ready to be Processed screen

When you click the **View Bills** link, your screen displays the Invoices, Unprinted, Non-CMS-1500s, as illustrated in Figure 4-13. The screen displays patients who have charges that have been posted and are ready for billing.

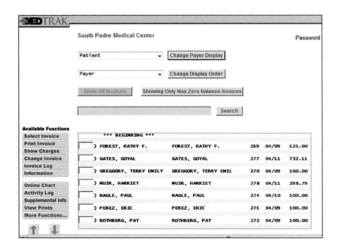

Figure 4-13: Invoice list view

Place your cursor in the command box next to FOREST, KATHY F and click the **Print Invoice** button on the left side of the screen. A heading will appear that states "Report sent to printer ..." When that prompt appears, click the **View Prints** button on the left side of the screen to go to the Available User Reports, where you will place your cursor again next to FOREST, KATHY F. Click the **View Report** on the left side of the screen. You are now at the Print screen, as shown in Figure 4-14. It is from this screen that you can print and save the invoice. Click the printer icon on the toolbar.

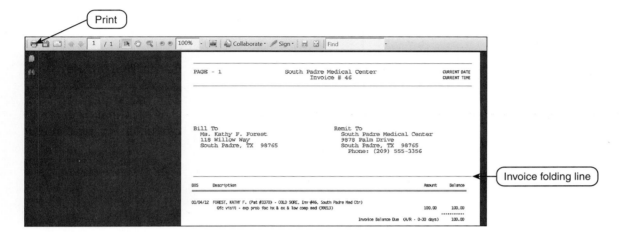

Figure 4-14: Print report screen

When the invoice prints, a single line will appear across the page under the "Bill To" and "Remit To" information. This line is provided to indicate where you will fold the page (see Figure 4-14) to allow the invoice to fit into a standard business windowed envelope. Figure 4-15 displays the invoice correctly folded, allowing the "Bill To" address to show through a window envelope. The top third of the invoice page is folded back, and the bottom third of the page is folded up.

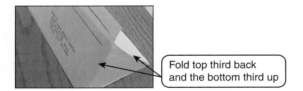

Figure 4-15: Folding an invoice

Figure 4-16: Windowed business envelope

DAY FOUR TASK 4.1

Gladys has directed you to print invoices for some patients who have charges posted.

From the Main Menu, click the **Billing** button. Next, click the **Bills to be Processed** button (center row). On the next screen, in the "Printed" section, place your cursor in the command box next to "Patient - Invoices" (see Figure 4-12) and click the **View bills** link on the left side of the screen. When you reach the Invoices, Unprinted, Non-CMS 1500s screen, place your cursor in the command box next to "GATES, GOYAL" and click the **Print Invoice** button on the left side of the screen. The report is sent to the printer, and you can access and print the invoice by clicking the **View Prints** button on the left side of the screen. Follow the same procedure used to prepare Goyal Gates' invoice for the remaining patients and save a copy of each in your Completed Work folder as follows:

1. Goyal Gates: LastName_YourFirstInitial_Task4.1Gates
2. Terry Emily Greggory: LastName_YourFirstInitial_Task4.1Greggory
3. Harriet Muir: LastName_YourFirstInitial_Task4.1Muir
4. Paul Nagle: LastName_YourFirstInitial_Task4.1Nagle
5. Eric Perez: LastName_YourFirstInitial_Task4.1Perez
6. Pat Rotherberg: LastName_YourFirstInitial_Task4.1Rotherberg
7. Tom Seyfer: LastName_YourFirstInitial_Task4.1Seyfer
8. Carol Smith: LastName_YourFirstInitial_Task4.1Smith
9. Norma Rae Wixo: LastName_YourFirstInitial_Task4.1Wixo

Task **4.2**

SCHEDULE PROOFING AND REVISIONS

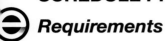

Requirements

- Access to MedTrak software

Gladys wants you to schedule Jason Eskew for an arthroscopic decompression of the left shoulder for Thursday, April 19, at 3 p.m. at the direction of Dr. Bond. There are already two separate blockings for that time on Dr. Bond's schedule—one for his surgery schedule and one for time when he is unavailable. Clear both blockings and enter the appointment for Jason Eskew and then reblock the remaining time in that day as "Unavailable." The appointment you added will display as in Figure 4-17. Save a copy of Dr. Bond's 04/19/12 schedule to your Completed Work folder as LastName_YourFirstInitial_Task4.2Bond12.

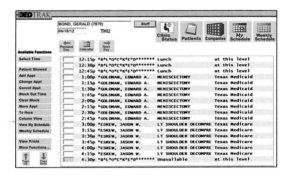

Figure 4-17: Jason Eskew's surgical procedure blocked on Dr. Bond's schedule

Gladys now wants you to do a check to ensure that any patients scheduled for a surgical procedure or return appointment have been properly scheduled. To do this, start at the Main Menu and click the **Patient Registration** button, which will display the patient database for the Center. Do a search for Eloise Fisher. Place your cursor in the command box to the left of Eloise Fisher's name and click **Appointments** on the left side of the screen. Your screen will display the appointments for Eloise as displayed in Figure 4-18.

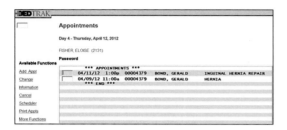

Figure 4-18: Eloise Fisher's appointments

Eloise had an appointment with Dr. Bond on Monday, 04/09/12, at 11 a.m. and is scheduled with him again on 04/11/12 at 1 p.m. Place your cursor in the 04/11/12 command box and click the **Scheduler** link on the left side of the screen. This link takes you to the Scheduling screen for 04/11/12 for the South Padre Medical Center. Change the Location to "Dr. Bond" and review Dr. Bond's schedule for 04/11/12. When you click the green down arrow to view the afternoon schedule, you will see that Eloise Fisher has been scheduled for an inguinal hernia repair at 1 p.m. that day. Click **Exit Screen** twice, and you will be back at the Appointment screen that displays Eloise Fisher's two appointments. Now, place your cursor in the command box next to the 04/09/12 appointment and click **Scheduler** on the left again, remembering to change the Scheduler view to Dr. Bond's schedule. Now you can verify that Eloise Fisher's appointment information is correct and that she was scheduled with Dr. Bond at 11 a.m. on 04/09/12.

You will start each search on the Patients screen, which you access from the Main Menu. The Patients screen contains the patients in the Center's database. For the following activity you do not have to go back and verify that the patient is on the physician's schedule as you did with Eloise Fisher; you only need to access the Appointment screen and verify that the appointments are listed correctly. Any appointment you see on the Appointment screen is already on the schedule because the information displayed on the Appointment screen comes directly from the schedules.

Exercise 4-1

Verify that the following appointments are listed as displayed on the Appointment screen for the patient. Correct any errors in the entries below.

1. Carol Smith
   04/09/12   10:30a   Bond, Gerald
   04/12/12   3:00p   Bond, Gerald

2. Terry Emily Greggory
   04/09/12   12:15p   Bond, Gerald
   04/11/12   1:00p   Bond, Gerald

3. William J. Foley
   04/09/12   1:00p   Bond, Gerald
   04/18/12   9:00a   Clark, Anthony

4. Jackie W. Masci
   04/09/12   4:10p   Adams, Ray
   04/12/12   2:45p   Clark, Anthony

5. Edward P. Goldman
   04/10/12   2:30p   Bond, Gerald
   04/19/12   1:00p   Bond, Gerald

6. Eugena Dore
   04/10/12   8:00a   Adams, Ray
   04/10/12   8:00a   Bond, Gerald

7. Jasper Hunt
   04/10/13   2:30p   Adams, Ray
   04/19/13   10:00a   Adams, Ray

8. Lori H. Whittaker
   04/11/12   8:00a   Adams, Ray
   04/11/12   2:00p   Bond, Gerald

9. Andi Andrews
   04/11/12   10:30a   Bond, Gerald
   04/20/12   1:00p   Bond, Gerald

10. Jason W. Eskew
    04/11/12   11:15a   Bond, Gerald
    04/19/12   3:00a   Bond, Gerald

11. Eloise Fisher
    04/10/12   11:00a   Bond, Gerald
    04/11/12   1:00p   Bond, Gerald

12. Harriet Muir
    04/11/12   5:00p   Harkness, Joyce
    04/12/12   12:00p   Harkness, Joyce

13. Floyd Barr
    05/11/12   8:00a   Harkness, Joyce
    04/11/12   11:00a   Harkness, Joyce

DAY FOUR TASK 4.2

Dr. Adams admitted Floyd Barr to the hospital at 10:25 p.m. on 04/10/12, but this was not an "appointment"—rather it was an "encounter," which is usually entered on the schedule as an appointment. Return to the patient database and locate Floyd Barr's name. In the command box, type "date" and hit **ENTER** on your keyboard. When you do this, you will see an encounter list for the patient, as displayed in Figure 4-19. There are only two appointments displayed—the 8 a.m. consultation and the 11 a.m. cardiac catheterization. The reason for this is that Dr. Harkness called the office and directed Gladys to place those two entries on her schedule. Most of the physicians bring papers to the office on which they have recorded the encounters they have had outside the Center (for instance, at the hospital). Other physicians call in these encounters to the office staff. Dr. Harkness often calls these encounters in and wants them placed on her schedule.

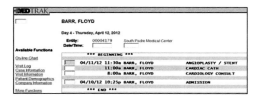

Figure 4-19: Encounters viewed from the Patients screen with "date" in the command box

The encounter record is a very useful feature because you can access many of the functions of the EHR from this screen, including the online patient charts. Place your cursor in the first command box on the Barr encounter record, which states "04/11/12, 11:30a Barr, Floyd, Angioplasty/Stent" and click **On-line Chart** on the left side of the screen. The chart will display, as shown in Figure 4-20.

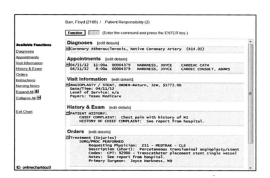

Figure 4-20: Floyd Barr's online chart

You will learn more about the online chart later; for now, click the **Exit Chart** link on the lower left side of the screen to return to the encounter list for Floyd Barr. With your cursor still in the command box beside the first Floyd Barr entry (04/11/12, 11:30a) on the encounter list, click the **Patient Demographics** link on the left side of the screen. The demographics (name, address, telephone number, etc.) appear on the screen, as illustrated in Figure 4-21.

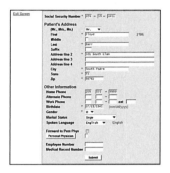

Figure 4-21: Floyd Barr's demographic information

Click the **Exit Screen** link on the left side of the patient demographics screen to return the Barr encounter list. With your cursor in the command box next to the 04/11/12, 11:30a encounter for Barr, click the **More Functions** link on the left side of the screen. Next, click in the box next to the term "Diagnosis" and then click the **Select Function** link on the left side of the screen. The diagnosis screen will display, as shown in Figure 4-22.

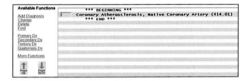

Figure 4-22: Floyd Barr's diagnosis for the angioplasty/stent service

From the diagnosis screen, you can add diagnoses, identifying them as the 1st (primary), 2nd (secondary), 3rd (tertiary), 4th (quaternary) diagnoses. Go back to the encounter list for Barr by clicking **Exit Screen** once. With your cursor in the command box next to the first entry (angioplasty) for Barr, click the **More Functions** link again. This time, click the box next to "Charges" in the list and then click the **Select Function** link on the left side of the screen. Your screen will display as in Figure 4-23.

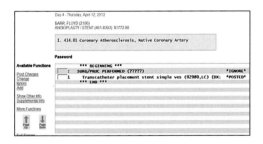

Figure 4-23: The CPT code and indication of "Posted"

This screen contains the CPT (service) code for Floyd Barr's transcatheter placement of a stent. Exit the screen and go back to the Main Menu. There is so much more to learn about the MedTrak system, and you will have the opportunity to do that in the days to come, but right now Gladys has some additional work for you to do. Gladys notices that Dr. Bond's schedule has been incorrectly matrixed to indicate that from 8-9 a.m. Dr. Bond is "Unavailable." Dr. Bond has rounds Thursday morning, so to correct this error Gladys asks you to remove

DAY FOUR TASK **4.2**

the blocking and replace it with 8:00-8:45 a.m. "Rounds" and 8:45-9:00 a.m. "Travel." When you are finished, make a copy of the 04/12/12 Bond schedule and save it in your Completed Work folder as LastName_YourFirstInitial_Task4.2Bond12.

Dr. Harkness calls the office to inform the staff that she has scheduled an 8 a.m. consultation at the hospital for Mathias Wellstone, a patient of Dr. Bethos. She has scheduled Mathias for a cardiac catheterization for 2 p.m. this afternoon based on a conversation she had with Dr. Bethos, who believes Mathias will require this procedure. Dr. Harkness wants you to record both of these encounters on her schedule for today. She is not going to conduct rounds at her usual time today, so you can remove that from her schedule and put the Mathias consultation in that time period. Dr. Harkness also states that she will not be returning to the office after performing the Wellstone catheterization; thus she requests that you block her time from 3-6 p.m. as "Unavailable." When you have finished with these revisions to Dr. Harkness' 04/12/12 schedule, save a copy in your Completed Work folder as LastName_YourFirstInitial_Task4.2Harkness.

Task **4.3**

ATTACHING DOCUMENTS

 Requirements

- Access to MedTrak software
- Patient Medical Documentation for Day 4, Task 4.3

Gladys has given you a list of medical documents that she wants you to attach to the patients' EHRs. The documents are located on the Evolve website in the Day 4, Task 4.3 folder. You previously uploaded documents to the EHR in Day 1, Task 1.3 and then subsequently on several other days of your internship. Refer to those directions for help with this task. Here are the documents you are to upload:

- Norma Rae Wixo, operative report, 04/11/12, Dr. Clark
- George Sorenson, operative report, 04/11/12, Dr. Harkness
- Steve Lopez, operative report, 04/11/12, Dr. Harkness
- Eloise Fisher, operative report, 04/11/12, Dr. Bond
- Lori Whittaker, emergency department report, 04/11/12, Dr. Sutton
- Lori Whittaker, radiology report, 04/11/12, Dr. Monson
- Lori Whittaker, orthopedic consultation, 04/11/12, Dr. Bond
- Lori Whittaker, operative report, 04/11/12, Dr. Bond
- Floyd Barr, cardiology consultation, 04/11/12, Dr. Harkness
- Floyd Barr, cardiac catheterization, 04/11/12, Dr. Harkness
- Floyd Barr, angioplasty/stenting, 04/11/12, Dr. Harkness

Exercise 4-2

Answer the following questions by referencing the documents you just uploaded to the patient's EHR.

1. Norma Rae Wixo's surgeon performed a treatment of the nasal bone with stabilization. Was the treatment open or closed? _____

2. The indications section of the cardiac catheterization for Steve Lopez stated that the procedure was performed due to what type of angina? _____

3. What type of anesthesia was used during Eloise Fisher's surgical procedure on 04/11/12? _____

4. Who was the attending physician when Dr. Bond performed Lori Whittaker's closed reduction? _____

Task **4.4**

INTERNET RESEARCH

 Requirements

- Access to MedTrak software

This morning Gladys has a special project for you. She asks you to use your computer skills to search the Internet for information on the keywords "Incident to." "Incident to" services are those that are furnished at the same time as the physician's professional service. Gladys specifically wants you to search for a government report that was prepared on the topic of "Incident to"; she recalls that the report number is SE0441. Do a search by typing "incident to SE0441 gov" in a search engine such as www.google.com or www.yahoo.com. Gladys says that this document, SE0441, is related to billing for Medicare patients. Locate the information using the search features of the Internet and save a copy to your Completed Work folder as LastName_YourFirstInitial_Task4.4Incidentto.

Next, you will assist Gladys with planning a meeting with the information you researched on "Incident to." The physicians requested the information on "Incident to" and would like Gladys to present the information at a meeting of all Center physicians. The meeting is to be scheduled for Wednesday, April 18, from 12 p.m. to 1 p.m. Gladys asks that you block 12-1 p.m. on all four physicians' schedules for Wednesday, April 18, with the reason as "Office Meeting, Incident to." Gladys explains that when she schedules a Center meeting, she uses the Center's primary location from which to schedule because it saves time and alerts everyone that there is a meeting. You are to access the Scheduler and book this meeting using the Location of "South Padre Med Ctr," rather than booking this meeting in each individual physician's schedule. Save a copy in your Completed Work folder as LastName_YourFirstInitial_Task4.4Meeting.

Well, that is the end of another busy day at the Center. Gladys continues to be very pleased with your work and sees that you are catching on very quickly to the process used at the Center and on the MedTrak system.

Just one final task before you are finished for this day—take the following short ten-question quiz.

Quiz

DAY 4

Using the MedTrak software, answer the following questions:

1. Which patient was scheduled for Dr. Harkness on 04/11/12 at 10 a.m.?
   a. Steven Lopez
   b. George Sorenson
   c. Harriet Muir
   d. Floyd Barr

2. Andy Andrews was scheduled for surgery on which date?
   a. 04/13/12
   b. 04/20/12
   c. 04/18/12
   d. 04/19/12

3. Accessing Floyd Barr's attached documents through the patient database and using the "doc" function, how many documents are currently attached to his charge?
   a. 0
   b. 3
   c. 4
   d. 6

4. How many documents are attached to Alice Cumming's EHR?
   a. 0
   b. 3
   c. 4
   d. 6

5. How many appointments are on the Gus Conrad appointment screen?
   a. 1
   b. 2
   c. 3
   d. 5

6. After clicking the **Billing** button from the Main Screen, which button on that Billing Menu screen will take you to the screen where you can post charges for services that have been provided by the physicians?
   a. Payment Batches
   b. Adj/Denial Batches
   c. Unbilled Dashboard
   d. Reminders

7. What patient is booked at 1 p.m. on Friday, 04/20/12, for surgery with Dr. Bond?
   a. Jason Eskew
   b. Eloise Fisher
   c. Lori Whittaker
   d. Andy Andrews

8. Using the patient database and the "date" function, what was the time of Jason Eskew's appointment on 04/11/12?
   a. 10:45 a.m.
   b. 11:15 a.m.
   c. 3:45 p.m.
   d. 8:00 a.m.

9. Using the patient database and the "doc" function, access Floyd Barr's attached documents and view the radiology report you attached to his EHR. What were the clinical symptoms indicated in the report?
   a. Chest pain, two view
   b. Chest pain, single view
   c. Chest pain, four view
   d. Chest pain, three view

10. Access Eugena Dore's attached documents and open the Emergency Department report. What was indicated as the chief complaint?
    a. Right hip pain
    b. Left hip pain
    c. Bilateral hip pain
    d. None of the above

It's time to receive credit for your quiz! Remember that you **must** go to the Scheduler, type "**QUIZ**" in any command line, and press **ENTER**. The next screen you will see displays a box that says "I am done with the Quiz for Day 4." If you are done, click **Yes**. If you have not completed the quiz, click **No** and you will be returned to the Scheduler. After you have clicked the **Yes** button on the Day 4 Quiz dialog box, your screen will display **Day 4 completed, Day 5 (April 13, 2012) charts loaded**.

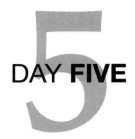

DAY FIVE

Friday, April 13, 2012

TASK **5.1**	Matrixing and Managing External Documents
TASK **5.2**	Inventory Management
TASK **5.3**	Scheduling Nursing Home Services
TASK **5.4**	Preparing Invoices

TASK **5.1**

MATRIXING AND MANAGING EXTERNAL DOCUMENTS

It is already the halfway point for your internship! You have learned so many things and have proven to be a most accomplished intern. All of the great skills you learned through your educational program are certainly paying off now. Keep up the good work and you will soon be finished with your internship and will have demonstrated proficiency in your chosen career.

Today, the center is closed and there will be no patients seen in the Center. The patient offices are being painted, and carpet is being installed throughout the Center. It is a good day to have this work done since three of the physicians were signed out for the day and Gladys cancelled Dr. Adams' patients. This type of day does not happen often in the Center, so everyone wants to make use of the time to catch up on unfinished tasks. Gladys has many things to do today and is glad that you are here to help her.

 First, Gladys wants you to remove the blocking from Dr. Adams' schedule for today and then reblock the entire day as "Unavailable." You do not need to save a copy of the schedule in your Completed Work folder. Next, Gladys wants you to upload medical documents to several patients' EHRs. Since you have performed this task many times during the week, she knows you can do it without direction. Upload the following documents to the EHRs:

1. Mathias Wellstone, cardiology consultation, Dr. Harkness, 04/12/12
2. Mathias Wellstone, cardiac catheterization, Dr. Harkness, 04/12/12
3. Mathias Wellstone, angioplasty/stenting, Dr. Harkness, 04/12/12
4. Harvey Clarkson, cardiac consultation, Dr. Harkness, 04/12/12
5. Bertha Wilson, cardiac consultation, Dr. Harkness, 04/12/12
6. Jean Olson, operative report, Dr. Clark, 04/12/12
7. Jean Olson, pathology report, Dr. Grey, 04/12/12
8. Dennis Dross, cardiac consultation, Dr. Harkness, 04/12/12
9. Terry Emily Greggory, operative report, Dr. Bond, 04/12/12
10. Carol Smith, operative report, Dr. Bond, 04/12/12
11. Harriet Muir, operative report, Dr. Bond, 04/12/12

Task 5.2

INVENTORY MANAGEMENT

Gladys has established an inventory system that is used throughout the Center to inventory equipment and furniture in excess of $50. Items less than $50 are not inventoried using the inventory process; rather, they are considered supplies. The inventory list contains the inventory number, product name, description, date purchased, and the room in which the item is located. Inventory updates are completed every 6 months in all rooms of the Center. Gladys assigns staff to various rooms in the Center, and those staff members submit a completed inventory form for the room(s) for which they are responsible. Gladys then uses a computer program to manage the inventory and prints a copy of the items in each room and distributes the copies to the responsible employee. The employee then determines that the equipment/furniture is in the assigned room and the inventory number is the same as is indicated on the equipment/furniture item. The inventory number is located on a tag that is glued to the back or underside of the item. To complete the Reception Inventory List in Figure 5-1, locate each item on the list in Figure 5-2; then write your initials in the dated column (far-right column). Your initials verify that the item is located in the room (displayed in Figure 5-2) and that the correct inventory number is located on the item.

South Padre Medical Center
Reception Inventory List

INVENTORY NUMBER	PRODUCT NAME	DESCRIPTION	DATE PURCHASED	ROOM	APRIL 13, 2012
RE1601	Normon	Reception Chair	01/15/XX	Reception	
RE1602	Normon	Reception Chair	01/15/XX	Reception	
RE1603	Normon	Reception Chair	01/15/XX	Reception	
RE1604	Normon	Reception Chair	01/15/XX	Reception	
RE1605	Normon	Reception Chair	01/15/XX	Reception	
RE1606	Normon	Reception Chair	01/15/XX	Reception	
RE1607	Normon	Reception Chair	01/15/XX	Reception	
RE1608	Normon	Reception Chair	01/15/XX	Reception	
RE1609	Normon	Reception Chair	01/15/XX	Reception	
RE1610	Normon	Reception Chair	01/15/XX	Reception	
RE1611	Normon	Reception Chair	01/15/XX	Reception	
RE1612	Normon	Reception Chair	01/15/XX	Reception	
RE6401	ThrillFlat	Table, round	08/03/XX	Reception	
RE6402	ThrillFlat	Table, round	08/03/XX	Reception	
RE6984	Swift	Stand, brochure	12/07/XX	Reception	
RE9021	Gabrial	Chair, child	03/06/XX	Reception	
RE9203	Swift	Picture, abstract	04/05/XX	Reception	
RE9204	Gabrial	Table, child	11/11/XX	Reception	
RE6111	Swift	Picture, abstract	01/04/XX	Reception	
RE6985	Normon	Rack, Magazine	01/15/XX	Reception	

Figure 5-1: Reception Inventory List

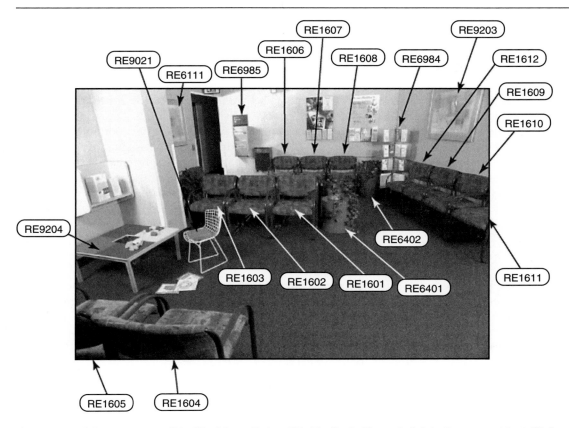

Figure 5-2: Office Inventory (Modified from Potter BP: *Medical office administration: a worktext*, St. Louis, 2010, Saunders.)

Task **5.3**

SCHEDULING NURSING HOME SERVICES

Once a month, Gladys schedules appointments for the physicians to see their patients at the South Padre Nursing Home. Today, Gladys will have you do the scheduling for the nursing home visits. Dr. Adams, Dr. Harkness, and Dr. Clark have stated that they would like to have a full morning or afternoon to go to the nursing home. If a full morning or afternoon is not available, schedule as much time as possible for the nursing home visits. The physicians have requested that they see patients at the nursing home on either Wednesday, April 18, or Thursday, April 19. The travel time will not be scheduled separately. For example, Dr. Harkness has lunch from 1-2 p.m., and 2-6 p.m. is marked off for the nursing home visit.

Dr. Adams prefers that you book his nursing home schedule on Wednesday, April 18.

- Save Dr. Adams' April 18 schedule as LastName_YourFirstInitial_Task5.3NSAdams

Dr. Harkness and Dr. Clark will not be in the office next week except for Wednesday, April 18, and they have asked you to matrix their schedules as "Unavailable" for Thursday, April 19, from 9:00 a.m. to 6:00 p.m. They want the nursing home scheduled on Wednesday, April 18.

- Save Dr. Harkness' April 19 schedule as LastName_YourFirstInitial_Task5.3Harkness19
- Save Dr. Clark's April 19 schedule as LastName_YourFirstInitial_Task5.3Clark19
- Save Dr. Harkness' April 18 schedule as LastName_YourFirstInitial_Task5.3NSHarkness18
- Save Dr. Clark's April 18 schedule as LastName_YourFirstInitial_Task5.3NSClark18

Dr. Bond prefers that you book his nursing home schedule on Thursday, April 19, from 9-12:00 p.m.

- Save Dr. Bond's April 19 schedule as LastName_YourFirstInitial_Task5.3NSBond

Task **5.4**

PREPARING INVOICES

Gladys wants you to process and prepare some invoices using the MedTrak system. Preparing invoices is a time-consuming and labor-intensive task, but the integrated MedTrak system makes the task so much easier. The software links the patient appointments to the accounting system and charges are automatically recorded after each appointment. When a service is rendered outside the Center (for instance, at the hospital), Gladys is responsible for creating a patient EHR and recording the services so that the appropriate invoice will be generated. She then uploads the documents that are sent by the outside facility to the patient's newly created EHR. You helped with this uploading task previously when you attached documents to the EHRs. It is now time to prepare the invoices for the patients who received services at the Center. Begin by opening the MedTrak system to the Main Menu. The first thing you must do is process the Unbilled Charges from Day 4 to ensure that the system will be up to date and ready to run current invoices. You have processed the Unbilled Charges before, so Gladys knows you can do it without direction. Be sure to process all the charges including commercial insurance, Medicaid/Medicare, and self-pay.

Once you have processed all Unbilled Charges from Day 4, the system is current. Go to the Main Menu and click the **Billing** button to display the Billing Menu screen that you accessed earlier to post patient charges. Today, click the **Bills to be Processed** button at the top of the second column. This screen is also one you have seen before—it displays the Printed and Electronically prepared bills areas. Today, we have 67 patients in the Printed, Insurance-CMS-1500 area of the Bills Ready to be Processed screen and one patient in the Patient-Invoice area. Place your cursor in the command box next to "Insurance-CMS-1500" and then click the **View Bills** link on the left side of the screen to display the screen in Figure 5-3.

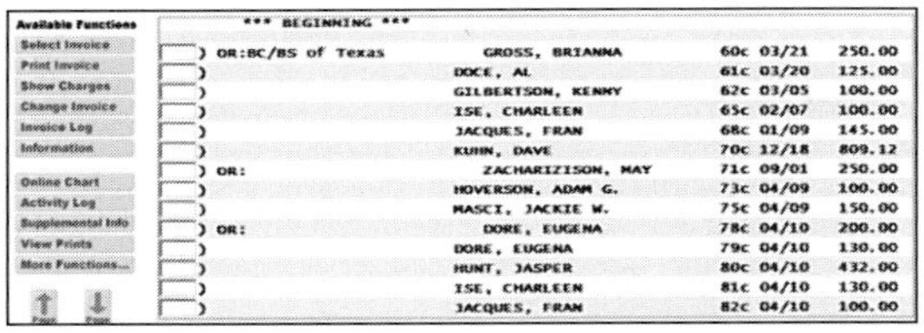

Figure 5-3: View bills screen

As displayed in Figure 5-4, use the drop-down arrow next to the Change Payer Display to change the order to All Payers and then click the **Change Payer Display** button to the right. Next, change the Change Display Order to Patient and click the **Change Display Order** button to the right. This step is very important because it ensures that the patients are in alphabetic order, which is necessary to correctly save the documents to your Completed Work folder.

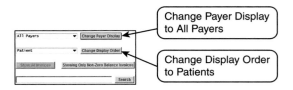

Figure 5-4: Changing display

The first patient in the list is Andy Andrews; place your cursor in the command box next to Andy Andrews and click **Print Invoice** on the left side of the screen. Your screen will indicate "Report sent to printer." Click the **View Prints** button and locate "...Andrews,_Andy_CMS-1500_Invoice...." on the Available User Reports screen. Place your cursor in the command box next to Andy Andrew's name. Click **View Report** and locate the CMS-1500 insurance form you just generated for Andy. Save a copy of Andy's insurance form to your Completed Work folder as LastName_YourFirstInitial_Task5.4Andrews.

Listed below and on the next two pages are the insurance forms you should save to your Completed Work folder and the names to use for each of the documents:

Andy Andrews	$125.00	LastName_YourFirstInitial_Task5.4Andrews
Floyd Barr	$225.00	LastName_YourFirstInitial_Task5.4Barr1
	$1,772.00	LastName_YourFirstInitial_Task5.4Barr2
	$1,942.00	LastName_YourFirstInitial_Task5.4Barr3
	$250.00	LastName_YourFirstInitial_Task5.4Barr4
Larry Bass	$75.00	LastName_YourFirstInitial_Task5.4Bass
Carol Blackman	$100.00	LastName_YourFirstInitial_Task5.4Blackman
Thomas R. Blair	$358.79	LastName_YourFirstInitial_Task5.4Blair
Mary L. Bogert	$100.00	LastName_YourFirstInitial_Task5.4Bogert
Ted Brown	$125.00	LastName_YourFirstInitial_Task5.4Brown
Harvey Clarkson	$1,942.00	LastName_YourFirstInitial_Task5.4Clarkson
Gus Conrad	$125.00	LastName_YourFirstInitial_Task5.4Conrad

DAY FIVE TASK 5.4

Alice Cummings	$125.00	LastName_YourFirstInitial_Task5.4Cummings1
	$183.00	LastName_YourFirstInitial_Task5.4Cummings2
Al Doce	$125.00	LastName_YourFirstInitial_Task5.4Doce1
	$125.00	LastName_YourFirstInitial_Task5.4Doce2
Eugena Dore	$130.00	LastName_YourFirstInitial_Task5.4Dore1
	$200.00	LastName_YourFirstInitial_Task5.4Dore2
	$2,362.00	LastName_YourFirstInitial_Task5.4Dore3
Dennis Dross	$1,942.00	LastName_YourFirstInitial_Task5.4Dross
Jason W. Eskew	$100.00	LastName_YourFirstInitial_Task5.4Eskew
Elizabeth M. Fenton	$150.00	LastName_YourFirstInitial_Task5.4Fenton
Norma Field	$257.50	LastName_YourFirstInitial_Task5.4Field
Eloise Fisher	$150.00	LastName_YourFirstInitial_Task5.4Fisher
Sandra Flannery	$194.00	LastName_YourFirstInitial_Task5.4Flannery
William J. Foley	$150.00	LastName_YourFirstInitial_Task5.4Foley
Amanda J. Foster	$100.00	LastName_YourFirstInitial_Task5.4Foster
Kenny Gilbertson	$100.00	LastName_YourFirstInitial_Task5.4Gilbertson
Edward A. Goldman	$150.00	LastName_YourFirstInitial_Task5.4Goldman
Nellie Groff	$125.00	LastName_YourFirstInitial_Task5.4Groff1
	$125.00	LastName_YourFirstInitial_Task5.4Groff2
Brianna Gross	$250.00	LastName_YourFirstInitial_Task5.4Gross1
	$249.00	LastName_YourFirstInitial_Task5.4Gross2
Adam G. Hoverson	$100.00	LastName_YourFirstInitial_Task5.4Hoverson
Maynard Hovlett	$250.00	LastName_YourFirstInitial_Task5.4Hovlett
Jasper Hunt	$432.00	LastName_YourFirstInitial_Task5.4Hunt
Gloria J. Hydorn	$160.00	LastName_YourFirstInitial_Task5.4Hydorn
Charleen Ise	$100.00	LastName_YourFirstInitial_Task5.4Ise1
	$130.00	LastName_YourFirstInitial_Task5.4Ise2
Fran Jacques	$145.00	LastName_YourFirstInitial_Task5.4Jacques1

	$100.00	LastName_YourFirstInitial_Task5.4Jacques2
Edna Jeffrey	$215.00	LastName_YourFirstInitial_Task5.4Jeffrey
Sylvia P. Kennedy	$125.00	LastName_YourFirstInitial_Task5.4Kennedy
Jackie L. King	$150.00	LastName_YourFirstInitial_Task5.4King
Josephine J. Knight	$125.00	LastName_YourFirstInitial_Task5.4Knight
Dave Kuhn	$809.12	LastName_YourFirstInitial_Task5.4Kuhn1
	$100.00	LastName_YourFirstInitial_Task5.4Kuhn2
Steven Lopez	$1,942.00	LastName_YourFirstInitial_Task5.4Lopez
Ramona Lorenz	$100.00	LastName_YourFirstInitial_Task5.4Lorenz
Jackie W. Masci	$150.00	LastName_YourFirstInitial_Task5.4Masci1
	$75.00	LastName_YourFirstInitial_Task5.4Masci2
Anne R. Meires	$100.00	LastName_YourFirstInitial_Task5.4Meires1
	$100.00	LastName_YourFirstInitial_Task5.4Meires2
David T. Oakland	$100.00	LastName_YourFirstInitial_Task5.4Oakland
Jean S. Olson	$4,289.00	LastName_YourFirstInitial_Task5.4Olson
Lewis L. Rock	$588.79	LastName_YourFirstInitial_Task5.4Rock
Silvia S. Scott	$150.00	LastName_YourFirstInitial_Task5.4Scott
Peter F. Silverman	$150.00	LastName_YourFirstInitial_Task5.4Silverman
George Sorenson	$1,119.00	LastName_YourFirstInitial_Task5.4Sorenson
Olivia Swen	$189.00	LastName_YourFirstInitial_Task5.4Swen
Mathias Wellstone	$700.00	LastName_YourFirstInitial_Task5.4Wellstone1
	$1,942.00	LastName_YourFirstInitial_Task5.4Wellstone2
	$1,306.85	LastName_YourFirstInitial_Task5.4Wellstone3
Greg Whitehead	$150.00	LastName_YourFirstInitial_Task5.4Whitehead
Lori H. Whittaker	$1,829.00	LastName_YourFirstInitial_Task5.4Whittaker1
	$200.00	LastName_YourFirstInitial_Task5.4Whittaker2
Maynard Zacharizison	$250.00	LastName_YourFirstInitial_Task5.4Zacharizison

When you have printed and saved the insurance forms for the patients listed above, click **Exit Screen** to return to the Bills to Be Processed screen. There is only one self-pay patient. Place your cursor in the command box next to "Patient-Invoices" and click **View Bills** on the left side of the screen. The Invoices, Unprinted, non-CMS-1500's screen displays only Bertha Wilson as a self-pay patient. Place your cursor in the command box next to Bertha's name and click the **Print Invoice** button on the left side of the screen. View the print you just made of Bertha's invoice and save it to your Completed Work folder as LastName_YourFirstInitial_Task5.4Wilson and exit to the Main Menu.

There is a function in the MedTrak system to batch all bills and run all CMS-1500 forms at one time. That is the function that Gladys uses; however, she wants you to run the CMS-1500s and invoices one at a time to ensure that you know how the system operates. The next time you run bills, you will use the batch function.

Gladys is very appreciative of your hard work today, especially the work you did on the invoices. That is a big job! You are done for another day, and it is the weekend already. See you on Monday to begin the last week of your internship.

You have just one final task before you are finished for this day—take the following short ten-question quiz.

Quiz

DAY 5

Using the MedTrak software, answer the following questions:

1. Upon accessing Mathias Wellstone's EHR, how many documents have been attached to his EHR?
   a. 1
   b. 2
   c. 3
   d. 4

2. When you access Harriet Muir's attached operative report, what is the pre/postoperative diagnosis?
   a. Tachybrady syndrome
   b. Tachybradia
   c. Tachycardia
   d. Angina

3. According to Dr. Adams' 04/16/12 appointment schedule, which patient is scheduled at 9:00 a.m.?
   a. Liz Furry
   b. Diana Morris
   c. Kenny Gilbertson
   d. Kin Zahn

4. According to Dr. Clark's 04/12/12 appointment schedule, which patient is scheduled at 2 p.m.?
   a. Jackie W. Masci
   b. Greg Whitehead
   c. Kenny Gilbertson
   d. Kin Zahn

5. From the Main Menu, which button would you click first to access the Billing Menu?
   a. Clinic Status
   b. Patient Registration
   c. Scheduler
   d. Billing

6. Once on the Billing Menu, you would click which button to access the accounts that need to be posted?
   a. Bills to be Processed
   b. Payment Batches
   c. Unbilled Dashboard
   d. AR Dashboard

7. When you use the "date" function with Andy Andrews, which of the following appointments is listed for Andy?
   a. 04/12/12
   b. 04/11/12
   c. 04/09/12
   d. 04/10/12

8. When you use the "date" function with Mary L. Bogert, which of the following appointments is listed for Mary?
   a. 04/12/12
   b. 04/11/12
   c. 04/09/12
   d. 04/10/12

9. When you prepared the CMS-1500 for Edward Goldman, what was listed on the form as the Total Charges?
   a. $250
   b. $150
   c. $325
   d. $125

10. When you prepared the CMS-1500 for Andy Andrews, what was listed on the form as the Total Charges?
    a. $250
    b. $150
    c. $325
    d. $125

It's time to receive credit for your quiz! Remember that you **must** go to the Scheduler, type "**QUIZ**" in any command line, and press **ENTER**. The next screen you will see displays a box that says "I am done with the Quiz for Day 5." If you are done, click **Yes**. If you have not completed the quiz, click **No** and you will be returned to the Scheduler. After you have clicked the **Yes** button on the Day 5 Quiz dialog box, your screen will display **Day 5 completed, Day 6 (April 16, 2012) charts loaded**.

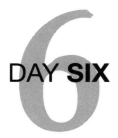

DAY SIX

Monday, April 16, 2012

TASK **6.1**	Arranging Physician Travel
TASK **6.2**	Responding to Telephone Messages
TASK **6.3**	Processing Pending Documents
TASK **6.4**	Patient Referrals

TASK **6.1**

ARRANGING PHYSICIAN TRAVEL

 Supplies Located on Evolve

- Travel schedule for Dr. Harkness

Gladys has supplied you with a handwritten itinerary from which you will prepare a travel schedule for Dr. Harkness' overnight trip. An example of the format you are to use to prepare Dr. Harkness' itinerary is displayed in Figure 6-1, A, and Figure 6-1, B is the handwritten itinerary. Once you have completed Dr. Harkness' itinerary, place it in your Completed Work folder as LastName_YourFirstInitial_Task6.1Harkness.

Itinerary for Dr. Joyce Harkness
New York City Cardiac Conference

4:45AM   **Friday, April 20, arrive at South Padre Airport**

5:30AM   **Flight 19 leaves South Padre destination New York City**

Figure 6-1, A: Travel schedule for Dr. Harkness

New York City Cardiac Conference

Dr. Harkness will leave Friday, April 20

Her flight is at 5:30AM

Needs to be at the airport at 4:45AM

Her flight # is 19

Non-stop flight from South Padre to New York City

Arrive in New York City at 9:00AM

Check-in New York City Hotel

Conference starts at 10:00am in the Green Room

Finishes at approx. 7:30PM

Leave New York City Saturday morning

Flight is at 7:30AM. Flight #229

Non-stop flight from New York City to South Padre

Be at airport at 6:45AM

Arrive at South Padre Airport at 12:00PM

****Reminder to Dr. Harkness to bring portfolio for conference and to pick up airline ticket at the check-in desk when she arrives at the airport.

Figure 6-1, B: Handwritten itinerary for Dr. Harkness

Task **6.2**

RESPONDING TO TELEPHONE MESSAGES

Supplies Located on Evolve

- Audio File Task 6.2

Some patients left "non-urgent" telephone messages over the weekend, and Gladys has asked that you listen to the messages (located on Evolve), record the pertinent information about each message, schedule appointments requested, and prepare messages in the MedTrak system. Gladys is going to work with you on this task because there are new functions to learn.

The first message is from a patient who wants an appointment with Dr. Bond for Wednesday, April 18. Log on to the MedTrak software and click the **Scheduler** button. Change the Location to Dr. Bond. Click **Calendar** to view the appointments for Dr. Bond for 04/18/12. The patient states that Dr. Andrews referred him to Dr. Bond, which makes this a referral (60 minutes). Place your cursor in the command box next to "9:00a" and click the **Add Appt** button on the left side of the screen. The patient database appears, but Mr. Johnson will not be in the database because he is a new patient. Click the **Add Patient** button on the left side of the screen and a Partial Patient Add dialog box appears. Enter the information for name (Johnson, Sven) and home phone (209-555-8881) and click **Submit**. The screen will flash and show the information you just entered, but you will also see a reconfirmation request to ensure that you really want to enter the information (see "Press ENTER to confirm" at the top of the dialog box). Click **ENTER** on your keyboard and your screen will display a request for the patient's payer information. Since you do not know whether the patient has insurance or not, click the **Self Pay** option and then click **Select Payer** on the left of the screen. The screen will flash and display "SELF PAY attached to patient ..." indicating that you have successfully identified the patient as a self-pay patient. Click the **Exit Screen** link on the left side of the screen. Place your cursor in the "P Self Pay" command box, indicating the primary payment is self-pay, and click **Confirm Payers** on the left side of the screen. You now will be on the Scheduling screen, which indicates that the patient is to be scheduled with Dr. Bond at 04/18/12 at 9 a.m.; you are to enter the reason (Lump on neck, Ref: Andrews) and the minutes (60) and click **Submit**. On the Appointment Note screen, type "None" in the highlighted box and click the **Submit Note** button on the left side of the screen. Mr. Johnson is now on Dr. Bond's schedule. Save a copy of Dr. Bond's April 18 schedule in your Completed Work folder as LastName_YourFirstInitial_Task 6.2Bond. You will need to call the patient to confirm the time and date of the appointment you reserved for him. When the patient presents to the office for the appointment, you will have him supply the necessary information about insurance, address, and other demographic data. Complete the short exercise below, based on the task you just completed.

Exercise 6-1

1. Below, write a draft of what you will say to Mr. Johnson when you call him to confirm his appointment with Dr. Bond.

_____

_____

_____

_____

_____

The second telephone message is from William Foley, who is a patient of Dr. Adams and Dr. Clark. From the Main Menu, click the Patient Registration button to open the patient database. Search for "Foley"; when his name appears at the top of the patient database list, place your cursor in the command box next to his name and click the **Appointments** button on the left side of the screen. The appointments list displays two appointments for Mr. Foley: 04/09/12 with Dr. Adams and 04/18/12 with Dr. Clark. Since today is 04/16/12, Mr. Foley has not seen Dr. Clark yet. You check the appointments to ensure that the patient has asked for the correct physician and has provided you with the correct appointment information. It is worth the extra step to check the appointments to ensure you are leaving an accurate message for the physician. Mr. Foley's question regarding laboratory information is referred to Dr. Adams. To do this, click **Exit Screen** on the left side of the screen to return to the patient database with William J. Foley's name on the top of the list. Place your cursor in the command box next to Mr. Foley's name and click the **More Functions** button on the left side of the screen. Click the box next to "Message" near the bottom of the More Functions list and click the **Select Function** link on the left side of the screen. A Further Review Needed dialog box appears, as illustrated in Figure 6-2.

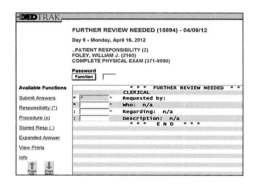

Figure 6-2: Further Review Needed

Note that the first command box is highlighted and your name follows "Requested by:" indicating that you are the staff member who is requesting a further review by the physician. Nothing more needs to be done to this "Requested by" information because it is automatically completed for you. Place your cursor in the second command box to highlight the "Who" line, which refers to the staff member who will receive the message on the Dashboard. You need the staff members initials for this box, so with your cursor in the "Who" command box, press the "F1" key on your keyboard (located at the very top left side of most keyboards). A list of initials for physicians and staff appears. This message is for Dr. Adams, so place your cursor in the check box next to his name and click the **Submit Selection** button on the left side of the screen. Now "RZA" appears next to the command box. Place your cursor in the Regarding box and type the patient's first initial and last name (W. Foley). Next, click in the command box next to the last line (Description) and click the **Expanded Answer** link on the left side of the screen. Type in the reason for the telephone call as "Wants lab results from Monday, April 9 office visit" and click **Submit Answer** on the left side of the screen. An asterisk will now appear in the fourth box, which indicates that the message has been stored.

Let's go find the message you just posted for Dr. Adams to view what he will see when he opens your message. Go back to the Main Menu and click the **Pending Menu** tab located at the top of the screen. On the Pending Menu, click the **Further Review Needed** button on the far right column. A Further Review Needed dialog box will open, as illustrated in Figure 6-3.

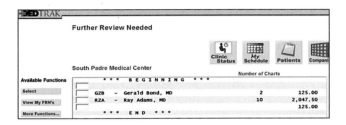

Figure 6-3: Further Review Needed

Place your cursor in the command box next to "RZA" and click **Select** on the left side of the screen. A new screen will appear with the items that Dr. Adams needs to review. You can see that Norma Field has some lab work that needs to be reviewed, but we are interested in the information for William J. Foley, so place your cursor in the command box next to "W. Foley" and click the **Show Order** button on the left side of the screen. When you do this, a new screen will open, as shown in Figure 6-4.

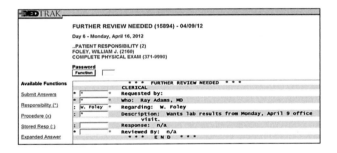

Figure 6-4: Further Review Needed for W. Foley

Note that there are lines for "Response" and "Reviewed By"—these allow the physician to type a response, enter his or her initials, and return the response to the sender. When you use this system, you not only send a message to a physician, but you also see where the message is stored and how the physician responds to requests for information. This system is a great advancement over paper telephone messages that can be misplaced or overlooked or may be difficult to read based on variations in handwriting. The electronic message remains in the query area until the message has a response from the physician. Exit back to the Main Menu.

The third message is from George Jones, who is a new patient being referred to Dr. Harkness. Following the same process you did for the earlier new patient, Sven Johnson, schedule an appointment for Mr. Jones. Gladys asks that you schedule the first hour-long appointment available on Dr. Harkness' schedule. Once you have placed the patient on Dr. Harkness' schedule, save a copy of her 04/18/12 schedule in your Completed Work folder as LastName_YourFirstInitial_Task6.2Harkness. Return to the Main Menu.

The last message is from Dr. Bond to his nurse. Gladys says that she will take care of this message for you because she is going to talk with Dr. Bond's nurse regarding another matter. She says that while she goes to talk with Dr. Bond's nurse, you can take your break and be back in 15 minutes.

Task **6.3**

PROCESSING PENDING DOCUMENTS

Supplies Located on Evolve

- Four laboratory results

Gladys wants you to learn how to process pending documents, specifically laboratory documentation. The courier service from Island Laboratories delivered some lab tests ordered by the Center's physicians for their patients. Download the laboratory results from the Evolve website for Day 6, Task 6.3. From the Main Menu, click the **Pending Menu** tab. From the Incomplete Visits area on the Pending screen, click the **Patient Responsibility** button. You will now see the Incomplete Patient Responsibility screen, which lists patient names and the type of incomplete information, as illustrated in Figure 6-5.

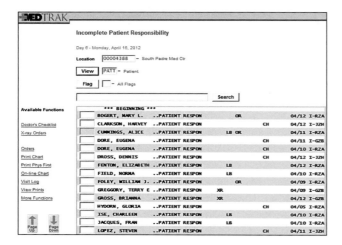

Figure 6-5: Incomplete Patient Responsibility screen

The meanings of the abbreviations in the center of the screen are as follows:

- OR = special orders
- LB = laboratory results
- XR = radiology reports
- CH = miscellaneous

Today, you are going to enter the "LB" information for the patients whose results you have received. The first patient with laboratory results is Alice Cummings. Place your cursor in the command box next to her name and click the **Orders** link on the left side of the screen to display the Visit Orders for Alice Cummings, as illustrated in Figure 6-6.

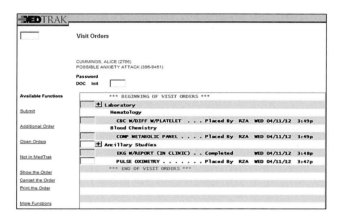

Figure 6-6: Visit Orders for Alice Cummings

Place your cursor in the blue command box next to "CBC W/DIFF W/PLATELET" and then click the **Show the Order** link on the left side of the screen to display the CBC order, as shown in Figure 6-7.

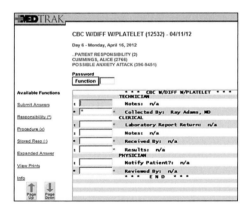

Figure 6-7: CBC orders for Alice Cummings

Note there are three main areas on the laboratory screen: TECHNICIAN, CLERICAL, and PHYSICIAN. The TECHNICIAN area indicates that Dr. Adams collected this sample for the CBC, which would usually be collected by a laboratory technician, but on this sample Dr. Adams obtained the sample himself. You will be completing the CLERICAL area. After you have completed the process, the physician will be notified that the laboratory results are available and that he or she can review and approve the results. Your part of this process is to indicate that the lab results are in and to upload the document to the patient record. So, let's get started with entering your information now. First, locate the copy of Alice Cummings' laboratory results and with the CBC screen open, place your cursor in the command box next to "Laboratory Report Returned" and type in "04/16/12." The items with a red asterisk following the box are mandatory to complete, whereas the boxes without red asterisks are optional. There are no "Notes" to enter for Alice's CBC, so skip that box, place your cursor in the command box next to "Received by," and enter your initials. Next, place your cursor in the "Results" command box and click the **Expanded Answer** link to display a yellow Notes box. In this box, type "See attached laboratory report dated 04/16/12," as shown in Figure 6-8. When you have entered the statement, click the **Submit Answer** button on the left side of the screen and you will be returned to the main screen for Alice's CBC.

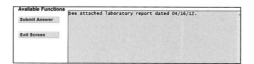

Figure 6-8: Expanded Answer screen for Alice Cummings

Alice also had "Comp Metabolic Panel" laboratory tests, so you will also need to process those results. Click **Exit Screen** to return to the Visit Orders screen. Place your cursor next to "Comp Metabolic Panel" and click the **Show the Order** link on the left again. The same three-section screen appears again for laboratory tests, so complete the CLERICAL section as you did for the other laboratory results. When finished, click **Exit Screen** to return to the Visit Orders screen. Alice also had Ancillary Studies of an EKG and Pulse Oximetry ordered, but those results are not back yet, so you cannot process those results. Click **Exit Screen** until you return to the other Incomplete Patient Responsibility screen. Elizabeth Fenton has laboratory results, so let's see what is pending for her. Place the cursor in the command box next to Elizabeth's name and click the link on the left for **Orders**. Place your cursor in the command box for the U/A and click **Show the Order**. When you do this, the laboratory results page will display (as in Figure 6-9), because this lab work was done in the center.

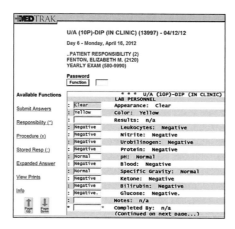

Figure 6-9: Laboratory analysis conducted in the center

When the laboratory work is completed by the Center laboratory technician, the technician enters the results directly into the computer and "flags" the physician that results are awaiting review. There is no Clerical section on the In Clinic laboratory report because nothing needs to be uploaded.

Click **Exit Screen** until you have returned to the Incomplete Patient Responsibility screen. Place your cursor in the command box next to Norma Field's name and click the **Orders** link on the left side of the screen. There are four serology results and one urine analysis. One at a time, place your cursor in the command box next to each laboratory analysis and enter the same information you did for Alice Cummings. You will see that the U/A DIP W/MICRO was conducted in the center, so you will not need to process those test results. Complete the processing for Charleen Ise and Fran Jacques; when done, return to the Main Menu for the final step in the process. You have already uploaded documents to patients' EHRs in the past, so Gladys asks you to please upload the laboratory documents as the final step in this assignment. Label the uploaded documents as "Lab Results."

Task **6.4**

PATIENT REFERRALS

Gladys has one more task for you before the end of this day. She would like you to learn about the referral process. Begin by opening the software to the Main Menu and clicking the **Pending Menu** tab. This is the same location from which you accessed the laboratory results to post charges, but instead of selecting the Patient Responsibility button, click the **Referral Dashboard** button. The Referral Dashboard contains three Pending patients, as displayed in Figure 6-10.

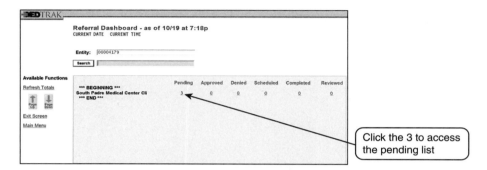

Figure 6-10: Referral Dashboard

Gladys wants you to process the three patients who are Pending on the Referral Dashboard. Under the Pending column head, click the **3** to display the three patients on the Referral Dashboard. The three patients listed are Larry Bass, Al Doce, and Paul Nagle. The reason for each referral is also listed-for example, Larry Bass is being referred to urology.

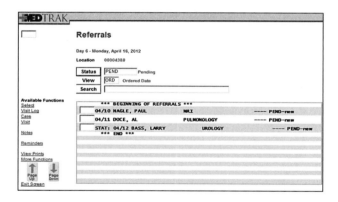

Figure 6-11: Referrals in the Pending category

The entry for Larry Bass is marked "STAT," which means the physician wants this patient's referral completed immediately, so we will process Larry's referral first. Place your cursor in the box next to his entry and click the **Select** link on the left side of the screen. A new screen opens, as displayed in Figure 6-12.

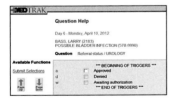

Figure 6-12: Referral request from Dr. Adams for Larry Bass

The Referral screen for Larry Bass indicates that Dr. Adams is referring the patient to a urologist for blood in the urine. Gladys states that because this was a STAT order, she has already called the urologist's office, Dr. Paula Smithson, and scheduled an appointment for April 30 at 3 p.m. Gladys points out that on the Urology screen, there are two areas: PHYSICIAN and CLERICAL. Dr. Adams has completed the PHYSICIAN area, which triggers the scheduling that you are doing now. Gladys explains that one of her responsibilities is to check on this Referral Dashboard several times a day and schedule any referrals that the physicians may have posted. It is the CLERICAL area that you will be completing today. It is important to note that there is more referral information than what appears on the screen. To view the remaining information, click the **Page Down** green arrow. Then click the **Page Up** arrow so that you are viewing the top of the referral information form. Also note that any block with a red asterisk following the block is mandatory information, whereas the blocks without red asterisks are optional information.

Place your cursor in the first CLERICAL box, "Referral status," which currently states "n/a" because there is no information stored in the system regarding the status of this referral. With your cursor in the "Referral status" box, click the **Stored Resp** link on the left side of the screen. A new screen displays three choices from which to choose, as shown in Figure 6-13.

Figure 6-13: Question Help in the Stored Response link

Gladys explains that because of the STAT nature of the referral, she has already obtained approval from Larry's insurance company for his referral to the urologist. Click the box next to "Approved" and then click the **Submit Selections** link on the left side of the screen. Your screen will flash and return you to the Referral screen, but now "Approved" appears twice: once in the "Referral status" box and again following "Referral status" within the line itself."

The next three lines on the referral screen are items that you would complete if you did not have approval on the referral, but since each of these has a red asterisk, we know we have to answer the questions. Place your cursor in the box next to "Referral step" and click **Stored Resp** on the left side of the screen. A new screen appears with a list of responses, as illustrated in Figure 6-14.

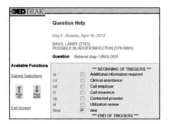

Figure 6-14: Referral step stored responses

The "Referral step" is asking you to identify what stage of the process the referral is in—for example, is additional information required or does the insurance company need to be called? Since Gladys already called and obtained approval, you can check the "new" box and then click the **Submit Selections** link on the left side of the screen. You will again be returned to the referral screen, where you can see that "new" is now in the block next to "Referral step" and "new" is also listed following the "Referral step" statement.

The "Referral notes" refer to any information that was provided to you regarding the referral; since there are none, key in "none" in the box and hit **ENTER** on your keyboard. When you do this, the word "none" will appear in the block and following the line "Referral notes" on the referral screen.

The "Reminder" is a function that you can enable if you are awaiting something in the referral process. The system will automatically remind you if there is information that you are awaiting before the referral process can be completed. Since we have approval for this referral, place your cursor in the box next to "Reminder" and click the **Stored Resp** link on the left side of the screen. A new box will appear with choices for No and Yes, as illustrated in Figure 6-15.

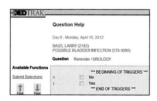

Figure 6-15: Stored responses for "Reminder"

Click the **No** check box and then click the **Submit Selections** link. The word "No" will then appear in the box and following the term "Reminder" on the screen.

The next line is for "Urologist"; this is used to indicate the physician to whom the patient is being referred. Place an "x" in the box next to "Urologist" and hit **ENTER** on your keyboard. A new screen will open, displaying the name of the urologist to whom the patients from the Center are referred, as illustrated in Figure 6-16.

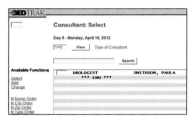

Figure 6-16: Selection of urologist from consultant list

Only one name appears on the list of urologists, but for other specialties there may be multiple physicians. Place your cursor in the box next to "UROLOGIST/SMITHSON, PAULA" and click the Select link on the left side of the screen. The screen then returns to the Referral screen, where you will see that Paula Smithson is now listed after "Urologist." Within the box there is now an asterisk, indicating that the physician to whom the patient is being referred has been selected.

The next line is the "Appointment Date"; Gladys made an appointment for Larry Bass with Dr. Smithson on April 30 at 3 p.m. Type "04/30/12" in the box next to "Appointment Date" and press **ENTER** on your keyboard. When you do this, your screen will flash and the date will appear in the Appointment Date box.

Place your cursor in the box next to "Appointment Time" and type in the time of the scheduled appointment. The format does not matter, because the time is only going to be displayed after the Appointment Time line. Thus you can type the time in a variety of ways ("3 p" or "3:00 pm" or "3 pm"). Type the time and then hit **ENTER** on your keyboard. The screen will again flash and the time will be displayed in the Appointment Time box and also after the Appointment Time line.

Gladys says that the patient needs to take a copy of the urinary analysis (UA) with him to the appointment with Dr. Smithson, so she wants you to place your cursor in the box next to "Medical Records" and click the **Stored Resp** link on the left side of the screen. The screen that opens (see Figure 6-17) allows you to check the box to indicate that the patient is to bring laboratory results to the referral appointment. Check the box now and then click **Submit Selections** on the left. Displayed on the Referral screen now is an asterisk, which indicates that you can read the entire statement by using the **Expanded Answer** link on the left. Place your cursor in the box next to "Medical Records" and click the **Expanded Answer** link to view the statement in the yellow box. If there were more directions that would fit on the referral page, you could click the **Expanded Answer** link to view that additional information. Click the **Exit Screen** button on the left and return to the Referral screen.

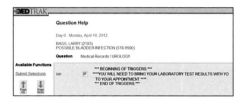

Figure 6-17: Medical Records for urology patient referrals

Once back to the Referral screen, click the green **Page Down** arrow to view the remainder of the referral form. There are three possible CLERICAL items yet to complete; also notice that the PHYSICIAN has one area to complete—reviewing the report from the consulting physician once the request report is returned to the Center from Dr. Smithson's office. Place your cursor in the box next to "Scheduling Clerk" and click the **Responsibility** link on the left to open the staff list. These are the people who have authority in the Center's system. Locate your initials, place a check mark in the box across from your initials, and then click the **Submit Selection** link on the left. From the Referral screen, you can also simply place your responsibility code in the box and hit **ENTER** on your keyboard. Either way, your name will now appear after the "Scheduling Clerk" and there will be a blue asterisk in the box, indicating that your name has been attached to this referral request. The remaining three blocks do not have to be completed by you. Although there is a mandatory indicator (red asterisk) on the "Consultation Summary," that is not a mandatory block to complete at this time, since the consultation has not taken place yet. Once the report is back from Dr. Smithson, you will go back to this form, indicate the date you received the report, and upload the document to the patient EHR. The physician will then be automatically notified that a report has come back for his patient, Larry Bass; at that point, he can review the report and then sign off on it by placing his responsibility code in the block next to "Reviewed By." However, for now, you have completed all the information required, so click **Exit Screen** once. Verify that there are no more "STAT" referrals that you need to process. Click **Exit Screen** once more. You are now back on the Referral Dashboard, and this screen needs to be refreshed to update. Do this by clicking **Refresh Totals** on the left side of the screen. Note that now "1*" appears in the Approved column. This is for Larry Bass, and the asterisk indicates that it is a STAT referral.

Gladys now wants you to click the 2 in the Pending column to see that you have yet to process Paul Nagle and Al Doce for referrals. Place your cursor in the box next to Paul Nagle and click **Select** on the left side of the screen. Gladys indicates that Mr. Nagle is to be referred to Dr. Argabright and that she has received approval from Paul's insurance company to refer him for the MRI. The scheduling priority (in the PHYSICIAN area) is indicated to be as soon as possible. Follow the same steps you used for Larry Bass, but this appointment time is 4 p.m. on 04/27/12. Gladys says there are no medical records that Paul will need to take to his appointment. Listed below is a shortened version of the directions you learned earlier:

- Referral status: Stored Resp link
- Referral step: Stored Resp (new)
- Referral notes: Key in None and hit **ENTER** on keyboard
- Reminder: Stored Resp link
- Location: Procedure link
- Appointment Date: mm/dd/yy and hit **ENTER** on keyboard
- Appointment Time: any format and hit **ENTER** on keyboard
- Medical Records: can leave blank or Stored Resp link
- Scheduling Clerk: Your Responsibility Code and hit **ENTER** on keyboard or Responsibility link
- Down Arrow
- Exit Screen
- Exit Screen again

After you click **Exit Screen** for the second time, you are returned to the Referral Dashboard. Notice that now a "1" appears in the Scheduled column (for Larry Bass) and a "1" in the Approved column (for Paul Nagle). This screen needs to be refreshed to update, so click **Refresh Totals** on the left side of the screen. After you have refreshed your screen, you should have "1" patient left in the Pending column. Click the **1** under Pending now.

The last patient who needs a referral for is Al Doce. Gladys has called his insurance company and received approval for an appointment with a pulmonologist (Gregory Dawson) on 04/25/12 at 9:30 a.m. Mr. Doce does not need to bring along any medical records to the appointment. Complete Mr. Doce's referral now. When you are finished, return to the Referral Dashboard, refresh your totals, and confirm that you have "3" patients in the Scheduled column. Access the referral page again by clicking the **3** under Scheduled, and you should see that the three patients you just scheduled for referral appear on the Referral screen. Place your cursor in the box next to "Paul Nagle" and click the **Select** link on the left side of the screen. You should now be back on the referral page for Mr. Nagle, where you can revise information if you need to. For now, click **Exit Screen** back to the Main Menu.

You now need to save a copy of the consultant letters. From the Main Menu, click the **Pending Menu** tab. Then click **Dashboard** under Referrals to go to the Referral Dashboard. Click the 3 under Scheduled to go to the Referrals screen. Place your cursor in the command box next to "Paul Nagle," type "PRCN," and hit **ENTER** on your keyboard. The Print/Fax Selection screen appears, as shown in Figure 6-18.

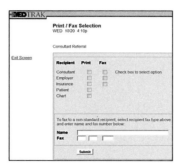

Figure 6-18: Print/Fax Selection screen

The options on this screen are Print and Fax. Choices of Recipient are Consultant, Employer, Insurance company, Patient, and Chart. Check the Consultant box under Print and then click Submit at the bottom of the dialog box. Do the same for Al Doce and Larry Bass. On the Referral screen, click View Prints and locate the three consultant letters you just printed; the patient's name and consultant referral will be in the document name. Save the three documents in your Completed Work folder as follows:

- Paul Nagle: LastName_YourFirstInitial_Task6.4Nagle
- Al Doce: LastName_YourFirstInitial_Task6.4Doce
- Larry Bass: LastName_YourFirstInitial_Task6.4Bass

You have just one final task before you are finished for this day—take the following short ten-question quiz.

Quiz

DAY 6

Using the MedTrak software, answer the following questions:

1. According to Dr. Harkness' itinerary, her flight number from New York City to South Padre is which of the following?
    a. 19
    b. 525
    c. 229
    d. 645

2. When a patient who is new to the Center is scheduled for an appointment via the telephone, you should do which of the following first?
    a. Add the name and telephone number(s) of the patient to create a partial patient
    b. Add the patient using the Add Appt button
    c. Confirm the payer(s)
    d. Add the name to create a partial patient

3. If you do not know the payer for a newly created patient, you should indicate which of the following as the payer?
    a. BC/BS
    b. Medicare/Medicaid
    c. Texas Health
    d. Self-pay

4. Which of the following is the first thing you should do when you return a telephone call to a patient?
    a. State your name and the name of the center
    b. Determine that it is the patient's residence, business, or cell and then state your name and leave the message with whomever answers the telephone
    c. Confirm to whom you are speaking; if it is not the patient, ask to speak to the patient
    d. State the name of your center and ask to speak to the patient

5. Which key on your keyboard do you press to display the initials of the physicians?
    a. F1
    b. F2
    c. F3
    d. F4

6. On the Incomplete Patient Responsibility screen, the abbreviation LB refers to which of the following results?
    a. Radiology
    b. Miscellaneous
    c. Special orders
    d. Laboratory results

7. Which of the following is not one of the three main areas on the laboratory screen?
    a. Technician
    b. Clerical
    c. Nursing
    d. Physician

8. If you were assigned to process the laboratory results that have been received from an outside laboratory, you would expect to also do which of the following tasks?
   a. Upload the results to the patient's EHR
   b. Key the laboratory results into the patient's EHR
   c. Either a or b
   d. Neither a nor b

9. When you access the Referral Dashboard and open Paul Nagle's referral form, you find that he is being referred to which physician?
   a. Gregory Dawson
   b. Paula Smithson
   c. Louis Argabright
   d. Ray Adams

10. When you access the Referral Dashboard and open Al Doce's referral form, you find that he is being referred to which physician?
   a. Gregory Dawson
   b. Paula Smithson
   c. Louis Argabright
   d. Ray Adams

It's time to receive credit for your quiz! Remember that you **must** go to the Scheduler, type "**QUIZ**" in any command line, and press **ENTER**. The next screen you will see displays a box that says "I am done with the Quiz for Day 6." If you are done, click **Yes**. If you have not completed the quiz, click **No** and you will be returned to the Scheduler. After you have clicked the **Yes** button on the Day 6 Quiz dialog box, your screen will display **Day 6 completed, Day 7 (April 17, 2012) charts loaded**.

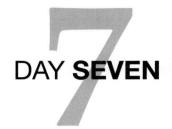

DAY **SEVEN**

Tuesday, April 17, 2012

TASK **7.1**	Personal Check and Credit Card Payments
TASK **7.2**	Insurance Company Payments
TASK **7.3**	Preparing Deposits

TASK **7.1**

PERSONAL CHECK AND CREDIT CARD PAYMENTS

Today, you will spend most of the day with Kerri Marshall, CPC, Insurance Specialist, and you will have an opportunity to learn about banking and deposits. Kerri has a batch of payments that arrived in this morning's mail, and she wants you to credit the payments to the correct invoice. The following are the payments:

- Bertha Wilson $ 50.00   Personal check #4569
- Norma Rae Wixo $ 686.00   Personal check #92934 for septoplasty
- Harriet Muir $ 98.79   Visa, Credit Card #4547890234, expiration date, 09/15 for office consultation (99242)
- Goyal Gates $ 25.00   Personal check #12563 for office visit, $125
- Carol Smith $ 20.00   Personal check #98235 for office visit
- Paul Nagle $ 62.00   Master Card, Credit Card #6980007001, expiration date, 11/14
- Pat Rothberg $ 50.00   Visa, Credit Card #5698759988, expiration date, 04/13
- Eric Perez $ 50.00   Personal check #45690

     TOTAL $1,041.79

DAY SEVEN TASK 7.1

Kerri explains that to post these payments, first go to the Main Menu of the MedTrak system and click the **Billing** button right above the "Near-time Wizard." Once on the Billing screen, click the **Payment Batches** button (left, second button from top). No batches have been generated at this point, so you will create one. From the Payment Batches screen, click the **Add** button on the left side to display the screen to create a new Payment Batch, as illustrated in Figure 7-1. The first blank to complete is the TIN (tax identification number). Key in "master" into the blank field and hit **TAB** on your keyboard. On the "Description" block enter "04/17/12 Your Initials"—thus if your name is Sue Ellen Jones, you enter "04/17/12 SEJ." Enter the Batch Total, or the amount of all the payments you will be entering today, which is $1,041.79—enter "1041.79" and then click the **Submit** button at the bottom of the dialog box.

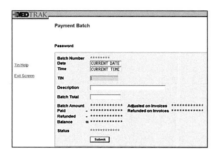

Figure 7-1: Payment Batch Add screen

The next screen is the Payment screen that will display the entry form for payments. The first payment was from Bertha Wilson, and her payment type was a check. Since the default is Check, there is nothing you need to do to the first blank.

The second blank is for the Source Type, which may be Patient, Private Insurance, Work Comp Insurance, or Other Payer. Click the Source Type down arrow to view the drop-down list, as illustrated in Figure 7-2. Select **Patient** as the Source Type. The TIN is already completed with the default MASTER.

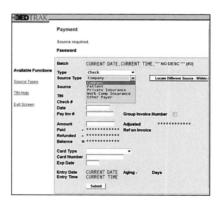

Figure 7-2: Changing the Source Type on the Payment screen

The check number for Bertha's payment is 4569. Key this number into the Check # block and then hit **TAB** on your keyboard to go to the next block. (Note: If you use the **ENTER** key, the patient database will appear because the **ENTER** function is the command to go to the patient database in the Payment Batch area. Use the **TAB** key rather than the **ENTER** key unless directed to do so in the directions.) Enter the Date as "04/17/12" and hit **TAB** on your keyboard. Tab through the Pay Inv # block and place your cursor in the Amount block. Enter the Amount for Bertha as "50" and then click **Submit** at the bottom of the dialog box. The patient database appears. Do a search for "Wilson" to display Bertha Wilson's name at the top of the list. Place your cursor in the box next to Bertha's name and click **Select Patient** on the left side of the screen. On the Invoices screen, which appears next, place your cursor in the box next to Bertha Wilson's name and click **Select Invoice** on the left side of the screen. The Payment Posting screen appears with the amount Paid highlighted. Enter the payment Bertha made ("50") and click the **Submit Payment** link on the left side of the screen. When you submit the payment, notice that Bertha's balance goes from 1942.00 to 1892.00, as illustrated in Figure 7-3. Since Bertha only has one charge, the payment will automatically be credited to that charge. If she had multiple services, you would have to indicate to which service the payment would be credited.

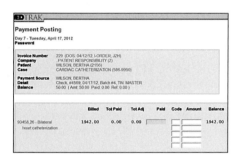

Figure 7-3: Payment Posting screen

Click the **Exit Screen** link on the left side of the screen, and the system will automatically return to the entry screen, where you can enter the next payment.

Kerri wants you to enter the personal payment from Norma Rae Wixo, but there is one thing she wants you to pay special attention to. At the Center, the invoice number is the number directly before the date of service. (The "c" next to the invoice number signifies that the invoice is in CMS-1500 format and is not part of the invoice number.) The number is automatically assigned by the MedTrak system each time invoices are produced. Kerri directs you to leave the Pay Inv # box blank when you fill out the payment for Norma because when you enter the amount and click **Submit**, you will be automatically directed to the patient database to select the patient account to which the payment is to be credited. When you select the patient and that patient has more than one service charge in the system, a screen will appear directing you to select the service that the payment is to be credited to. For example, when you place your cursor in the command box next to Norma's name and click the **Select Invoice** button on the left side of the screen, you are returned to the Payment Posting screen. You will see that Norma has two charges, and you need to assign the payment to either one or both charges. Norma has indicated that she wants the payment to be applied to the septoplasty charge, so type the total check amount as "686.00" in the box under the Paid heading and hit **ENTER** on your keyboard. The Payment Posting screen will flash and display the new totals after crediting the amount to the septoplasty charge. Click **Exit Screen** on the left side of the screen. You will see a message on the top of the screen that indicates "Successful add - ready to add another..."

The next patient made a payment using a credit card. From the Type drop-down menu, select **Credit card** as illustrated in Figure 7-4.

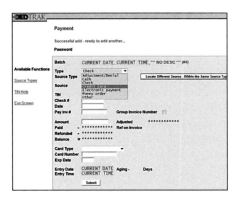

Figure 7-4: Preparing to record a credit card payment

Change the Source Type to **Patient**. Tab forward to the Date block and enter "04/17/12." Place your cursor in the Pay Inv # block and hit **ENTER** on your keyboard to display the patient database. Do a search for "Muir" to display Harriet Muir's name at the top of the list. Place your cursor in the box next to Harriet's name and click **Select Patient** on the left side of the screen. The screen defaults to the Amount box, where you type "98.79" and hit **ENTER** on your keyboard. The screen defaults to Card Type, where you click the drop-down arrow and select **Visa**. Place your cursor in the Card Number box and key in "4547890234"; then place your cursor in the Exp Date box, enter "09/15," and click **Submit** at the bottom of the dialog box. The Invoices screen appears, where you place your cursor in the command box next to Harriet's name and click **Select Invoice** on the left side of the screen. Harriet indicated she wanted the total payment to be credited to the office consultation (99242). Type "98.79" in the first block under Paid and hit **ENTER** on your keyboard. When you do this, note that the screen updates to reflect the payment and also the top of the page indicates that the patient made a Visa credit card payment for 98.79, as illustrated in Figure 7-5.

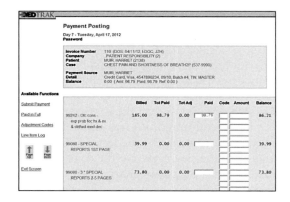

Figure 7-5: Payment Posting for Harriet Muir

Kerri wants you to record the three personal checks that remain. She also provides you with the following shorter version of the directions for personal checks:

- Begin on Payment screen
- **Type:** Keep default Check
- **Source Type:** Change to Patient
- **Check #:** Enter check #; then hit TAB
- **Date:** Key in as mm/dd/yy
- **Pay Inv #:** Leave blank
- **Amount:** Enter amount and hit **Submit**
  - Patient Status, cursor next to patient, Select Patient
  - Invoices screen, cursor next to patient, Select Invoice
  - Type amount under Paid; then hit **ENTER**
  - Verify amount correct, check correct
- **Exit Screen:** Return to next patient

Once you have entered all the personal checks, enter the credit card payments. When you have entered all of the payments in this batch, you will save a copy in your Completed Work folder. To save a copy of the batch you just created, go to the Main Menu, click **Billing**, then click **Payment Batches**, and then click the **Showing all balances** button above the box where you would enter a search term. Your screen will display as in Figure 7-6.

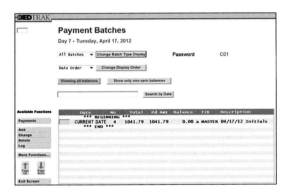

Figure 7-6: Payment Batches screen

Place your cursor in the box next to the batch you just created and click the **More Functions** button on the left side of the screen. A dialog box will open and you will check the box next to "Print Payments in Batch," as illustrated in Figure 7-7.

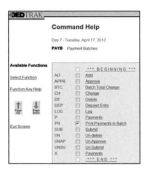

Figure 7-7: Printing Payment Batch

With the "Print Payments in Batch" box checked, click the Select Function link on the left side of the screen. You will be returned to the Payment Batch screen, where you will click Exit Screen until you see View Prints located on the top left hand corner of the screen. When you open the View Prints window, your document will have "Payment_Batch_Report" in the title. Save a copy of the report to your Completed Work folder as LastName_YourFirstInitial_Task7.1Batch1. Kerri also asks that you print a copy of the batch to be used in preparation of a bank deposit ticket that you will be completing at the end of the day.

Exercise 7-1

1. What was the payment amount Bertha Wilson made by personal check? _____

2. What was the expiration date on Harriet Muir's credit card? _____

3. What credit card did Pat Rothberg use for her account payment? _____

4. For what procedure did Norma Rae Wixo make a payment? _____

Task 7.2

INSURANCE COMPANY PAYMENTS

Kerri received two insurance checks and would like for you to learn how to apply the payments to the individual patient accounts. The first is check # 560923 from Texas Health Corporation, 2702 Oak Line Drive, South Padre, TX 98765, in the amount of $1,899.

Patient	Charge	Payment	Adjustment
Andy Andrews	125	110	15
Larry Bass	75	55	20
Ted Brown	125	100	25
Harvey Clarkson	1942	1422	520
Gus Conrad	125	100	25
Jackie L. King	150	112	38
TOTALS	**2542**	**1899**	**643**

From the Main Menu, click **Billing** and then **Payment Batches**. Click the **Add** button on the left to display the screen where you will create a Payment Batch. The information for the screen is as follows:

TIN: Master
Description: TxHealthCorp 04/17/12 Your Initials
Batch Total: 1899
Submit

On the Payment screen, the entry information is as follows:

Type: Check
Source Type: Private Insurance
Check #:   560923
Date: 04/17/12
Pay Inv #:   Blank
Amount: 110
Submit

The Entity/Payer: Select screen appears; click in the command box next to "Texas Health Corporation" and click **Select Payer** from the left side of the screen. The Invoices screen appears, and you will do a search for "Andrews" and then hit **ENTER**. The invoices are sorted, and Andy Andrews appears on the top of the list. Place your cursor in the command box in front of Andy's name and click the **Select Invoice** button from the left side of the screen.

The Payment Posting screen appears with the Invoice Number on top, along with the company, patient, and case information in green and below that the Payment Source, Detail, and Balance in blue, as illustrated in Figure 7-8.

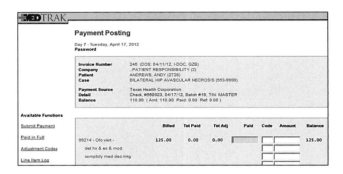

Figure 7-8: Payment Posting

The default highlighted area is the Paid block, where you type the amount the insurance company paid on the service. Then hit **TAB** until you get to the Code column. From here, you can click the **Adjustment Codes** link on the left to display the list of adjustment, or you can type "A01" in the Code column and enter the amount of the adjustment in the Amount column. Then hit **ENTER** on your keyboard. The numbers you just entered will become blue, and the balance column on the far right will be 0.00, indicating you have successfully entered the payment. Since the last **ENTER** submitted the payment, you now click the **Exit Screen** link on the left side of the screen to be returned to the Invoices list, where you can locate the next patient and continue posting the remaining payments.

When you have entered the last patient and the balance left in the check amount is 0, you will be returned to the Payment Batches screen to create another payment batch. However, you need to print the batch you just created, so click **Exit Screen** on the left side of the screen. Continue clicking **Exit Screen** until you are back to the Payment Batches screen. Click the **Showing all Batches** button and you will see the date you created the batch and the total amount of the check (1899.00), the paid amount applied to invoices (1899.00), the balance to be applied (0.00), and the description (TxHealthCorp). To print the batch payment, place your cursor next to the batch you just created, click the **More Functions** button, select **Print Payments in Batch** from the list, and click **Select Function**. Again, you will not see the View Prints button on this screen, so exit the screen twice to get to the Billing Menu, where you can click the **View Prints** button. Locate the batch print and save a copy to your Completed Work folder as LastName_YourFirstInitial_Task7.2Batch2. Kerri also asks that you print a copy of the batch to be used in preparation of a bank deposit ticket that you will be completing at the end of the day.

Kerri has another check from Texas Medicare for which she wants you to create a payment batch. She provides you with the following information:

Name of batch: TxMed 04/17/12
Amount of check: $3,436
Check #: 67502145

Patient	Charge	Payment	Adjustment
Floyd Barr	225	210	15
Floyd Barr	1772	1572	200
Floyd Barr	1942	980	962
Floyd Barr	250	200	50
Jason W. Eskew	100	64	35
Elizabeth M. Fenton*	150	100	38
	130	90	40
	20	10	10
Norma Field*	257	190	
	140	138	2
	97.50	42	55.50
	20	10	10
Sandra Flannery*	194	120	
	125	70	55
	69	50	19
TOTALS	**4890**	**3436**	**1454.50**

*Patient has invoice for first column amount; on invoice details, amounts are as shown.

When you have completed the entry, save a copy of the batch to your Completed Work folder as LastName_YourFirstInitial_Task7.2Batch3. Kerri also asks that you print a copy of the batch to be used in preparation of a bank deposit ticket that you will be completing at the end of the day.

Kerri provides you with these written steps to create a batch payment:

- Main Menu
- Billing
- Payment Batches
  - Add
  - Master
  - Description: TxMed 04/17/12 Your Initials
  - Check: 3436 (batch total)
  - Submit
- **Payment Screen**
  - Type: Check
  - Source Type: Private Insurance
  - Check #: 67502145
  - Date: 04/17/12
  - Pay Inv #: Blank
  - Amount: Individual patient payment
  - Submit
- **Entity/Payers: Select**
  - Check Texas Medicare
  - Select **Payer** link
  - **Invoices**
  - Search for patient
  - Cursor in command box; select **Invoice**
  - Paid: Amount paid + **TAB**
  - Code: A01 for adjustment
  - Amount: Adjustment amount + **ENTER**
  - Proof entry
  - **Exit Screen** and print
  - **Exit Screen** to Billing Menu to **View Prints**
- Repeat

Task **7.3**

PREPARING DEPOSITS

 Supplies Located on Evolve

- Deposit Ticket

Kerri has asked that you complete the deposit ticket for the checks received today. You have copies of the payment batches saved in your Completed Work folder and you also printed a copy of the three batches. Referring to the documents for the three batches you created, begin to enter the checks on the deposit ticket you downloaded from the Evolve website.

First, though, Kerri wants you to go to the Main Menu, Billing, and Payment Batches. Once on the Payment Batches screen, click the **Showing all balances** button at the top of the page. When you do this, the three batches that you created today will be displayed:

> $1,041.79, Batch 1, personal checks and credit card
>
> $1,899.00, Batch 2, Texas Health Corporation
>
> $3,436.00, Batch 3, Texas Medicare

Total: $6,376.79

There were three credit card payments of $210.79 in Batch 1, for a total of deposits of $6,166 for the day.

Complete the deposit ticket by entering one check on each line. For example, you will type "Wilson" and check number "4569" for $50.00, as illustrated in Figure 7-9.

DEPOSIT TICKET

SOUTH PADRE MEDICAL CENTER
9878 PALM DRIVE
SOUTH PADRE, TX 98765

FIRST NATIONAL BANK
100 FIRST STREET
SOUTH PADRE, TX 98765

DATE _____
DEPOSITS MAY NOT BE AVAILABLE FOR IMMEDIATE WITHDRAWAL

		DOLLARS	CENTS
CURRENCY			
COIN			
CHECKS LIST EACH SEPARATELY			
1 Wilson	4569	50	00
2			
3			
4			

Figure 7-9: Deposit ticket entry format

Since there are only seven entries, you can use one block per entry. Once you have entered the seven checks, type the total in the TOTAL area at the bottom of the deposit ticket and also in the grey box that runs sideways on the left side of the deposit ticket.

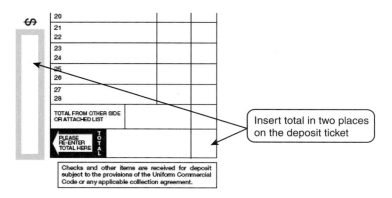

Figure 7-10: Deposit ticket totals

Enter the date on the deposit ticket as "04/17/12."

Exercise 7-2

1. What is the total of the deposit ticket you just completed? _____

2. What was the total of the Texas Health Corporation check? _____

3. How many checks were on the deposit ticket? _____

4. How many batches did you create today? _____

Kerri is very pleased that you have completed the payment tasks; she appreciates your hard work in accomplishing the tasks she gave you. She shares with Gladys how quickly you caught on to the payment process and says she looks forward to having you back.

You have just one final task before you are finished for this day—take the following short ten-question quiz.

Quiz

DAY 7

Using the MedTrak software, answer the following questions:

1. Norma Rae Wixo wrote a personal check for _____ that you posted on 04/17/12.
   a. $50
   b. $25
   c. $98.79
   d. $686.00

2. What is the TIN number for the Center?
   a. Center
   b. Clinic
   c. Padre
   d. Master

3. Texas Health Corporation sent the Center a check for _____ that you deposited on 04/17/12.
   a. $2,542
   b. $1,899
   c. $4,890
   d. $3,436

4. Texas Medicare sent the Center a check for _____ that you deposited on 04/17/12.
   a. $2,542
   b. $1,899
   c. $4,890
   d. $3,436

5. What was the amount of the deposit you completed on 04/17/12?
   a. $6,166
   b. $6,661
   c. $6,427
   d. $6,966

6. To access the Payment Batch screen to create a new batch from the Main Menu of the MedTrak system, you would follow which path?
   a. Patient Registration, Patient, Select Invoice, Payment Batch
   b. Administration, Billing, Payment Batch
   c. Billing, Payment Batches, Add
   d. None of the above

7. What is the three-digit code you place in the Payment Posting Code column to indicate an adjustment was made to the payment by the insurance company?
   a. A10
   b. A11
   c. A00
   d. A01

8. When you are on the Payment Batches screen, you click which button to display the batches you created today?
   a. Change Batch Type Display
   b. Showing all balances
   c. Change Display Order
   d. Show only non-zero balances

9. On the Payment Batches screen with your three batches displayed on your screen, place your cursor in the Texas Health Corporation batch, and click the Change button. What is the amount of the adjustment made on the invoices?
   a. 643
   b. 644
   c. 633
   d. 634

10. On the Payment Batches screen with your three batches displayed on your screen, place your cursor in the Texas Medicare batch, and click the Change button. What is the amount of the adjustment made on the invoices?
    a. 1544
    b. 1454.50
    c. 1455
    d. 1455.50

It's time to receive credit for your quiz! Remember that you **must** go to the Scheduler, type "**QUIZ**" in any command line, and press **ENTER**. The next screen you will see displays a box that says "I am done with the Quiz for Day 7." If you are done, click **Yes**. If you have not completed the quiz, click **No** and you will be returned to the Scheduler. After you have clicked the **Yes** button on the Day 7 Quiz dialog box, your screen will display **Day 7 completed, Day 8 (April 17, 2012) charts loaded**.

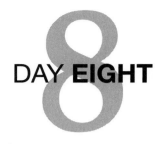

DAY EIGHT

Wednesday, April 18, 2012

TASK 8.1

ADDING PATIENTS TO THE DATABASE

Today, you will work at the front desk with Gladys. There are always many walk-in patients at the Center, and Gladys is going to show you how to register these patients.

The first walk-in patient is Dianne G. Barron. She presents to the desk and would like to see a physician for a headache. Gladys tells the patient that Dr. Adams can see her today at 10 a.m. and asks Dianne to complete a patient information form; the patient completes the form and returns it to the front desk. Gladys wants you to enter Dianne in the patient database. When you do this, the patient is automatically registered in the MedTrak system and recognized as a patient waiting in the waiting room to see a physician.

Beginning at the Main Menu, click the **Patient Registration** button and then click the **Add Patient** button on the left side of the screen. The first screen is Patient: Add by SSN, as illustrated in Figure 8-1. Dianne's Social Security number is **261-44-0022**. Enter her SSN and click the **Submit** button at the bottom of the dialog box.

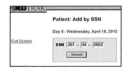

Figure 8-1: Adding a patient to the patient database

DAY EIGHT TASK 8.1

The Patient screen, as displayed in Figure 8-2, will appear after you submit the SSN. This screen is where you input the patient demographic information.

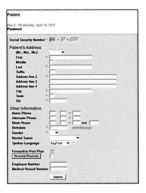

Figure 8-2: Patient demographic information

Enter this information in the appropriate fields on the patient demographic screen for Dianne:

Name:	**Ms. Dianne G. Barron**
Address:	**508 Clam**
	South Padre, TX 98765
Home Telephone:	**209-555-2095**
Birthdate:	**09/07/1939**
Gender:	**Female**
Marital Status:	**Single**

Once you have entered all the data, click **Submit**. As illustrated in Figure 8-3, the screen flashes and reappears to give you an opportunity to review the information for correctness. If any information you input is incorrect, press **F3** (top left of your keyboard); if everything is correct, press **ENTER** on the keyboard. When you have proofed the information and verified that it is accurate, press **ENTER** to move on to the Companies screen.

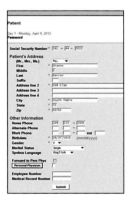

Figure 8-3: Reviewing patient demographic information

Companies screen

Dianne has no insurance, so she is a self-pay patient. Place your cursor in the command box next to "Patient responsibility" (Figure 8-4). Click **Select Company** on the left side of screen to go to the next screen, which is the New Case screen.

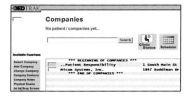

Figure 8-4: Selecting the payer

New Case screen

The New Case screen is where the patient's complaint is recorded, as illustrated in Figure 8-5.

Complaint: Headache

Click **Submit** to move on to identify the Entity/Payers.

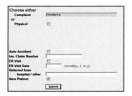

Figure 8-5: Indicating the complaint or physical

Entity/Payers: Select screen

The Entity/Payers: Select screen is where you confirm the payer you previously identified (Figure 8-6). Click the command box next to "Self Pay" and then click **Select Payer** on the left side of the screen.

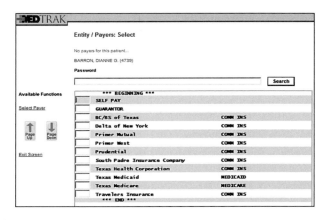

Figure 8-6: Indicating the Payer

The Entity/Payers: Select screen will reappear, this time indicating "Self Pay attached to patient" above the patient's name, as illustrated in Figure 8-7. Click **Exit Screen**.

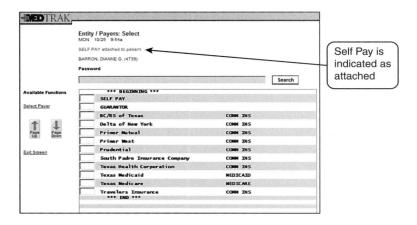

Figure 8-7: Self Pay attached confirmed

The Patient/Payers screen indicates that the patient's primary payment method is self-pay. Note the "P" next to "Self Pay," which indicates "Primary" (Figure 8-8). It is on this screen that you can indicate another payer or change the self-pay from primary to secondary, etc. Place your cursor in the box next to "P Self Pay" and click **Confirm Payers** on the left side of the screen.

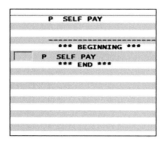

Figure 8-8: Confirming Self Pay

Visit Add screen

The Visit Add screen is where you indicate the type of visit (Figure 8-9). Click the arrow in the box next to "Type of Visit" and from the drop-down menu, select **Doctor** and click **Submit**.

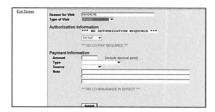

Figure 8-9: Visit Add screen

Nursing Note Add screen

The Nursing Note Add screen appears next; check "Headache" on the list by clicking the box next to that entry, as illustrated in Figure 8-10. Click **Submit**.

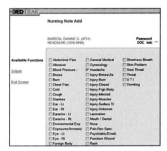

Figure 8-10: Nursing Note Add screen with "Headache" checked

The Nursing Note Add screen appears again to allow for additional complaints to be added, but since this patient only had the complaint of headache, click **Exit Screen** to return to the Patients screen, as shown in Figure 8-11. Hit **ENTER** on you keyboard to process the changes. Dianne G. Barron is now registered in the Center's database.

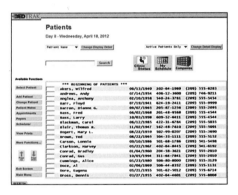

Figure 8-11: Dianne Barron listed in the patient database

Gladys asks you to go to the Main Menu and click the **Clinic Status** button to see where Dianne has been placed within the MedTrak system. Figure 8-12 shows that Dianne is waiting for a room, which is indicated by the word "Room" in green type in the Status column. In the column labeled "TC," which stands for "medical technician, medical assistant, nurse," is the amount of time Dianne has been in the waiting room. When the nursing staff calls the patient from the waiting room into a patient examination room, the time is recorded in the MedTrak system. Once the physician goes into the examination room to see that patient, the DR column begins to track the time the physician spends with the patient. When the physician has finished with the examination, he or she indicates the ending time within the MedTrak system. Wherever the patient goes within the Center, the Clinic Status screen tracks the patient. Since the staff will not be managing the patient once you enter the patient's information in the system, the patient will continue to appear to be waiting for a room. Return to the Main Menu.

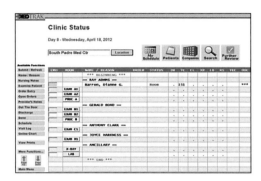

Figure 8-12: Patient registered and awaiting Dr. Adams

Another patient has arrived as a walk-in with a chief complaint of sprained right ankle. Gladys directs you to register the patient. The patient has provided you with the following information:

SSN:	**501-66-1110**
Name:	**Mark Bogert**
Address:	**2502 32nd Avenue South**
	South Padre, TX 98765
Home Telephone:	**209-555-3690**
DOB:	**09/12/1959**
Gender:	**Male**
Marital Status:	**Married**

Click **Submit**.
Press **ENTER** if correct or **F3** to change.

Companies

Click **Patient Responsibility**.
Select **Company**.

New Case

Complaint: **Sprained right ankle**

Click **Submit**.

Entity/Payers: Select

Insurance: **South Padre Insurance Company**

Click **Select Payer**.

Patient/Payer

Subscriber Relationship: **Self**
Last Name: **Bogert**
First Name: **Mark**
Middle Initial: Leave blank
DOB: **09/12/1959**
Gender: **Male**
Effective: **01/10/08**
Term Date: Leave blank
ID #   **MNY2691**
Group Name: **Partners**
Group #:   **40005**
Plan Type: **Basic Health**
Co-Insurance %:   **20%**
Co-Pay Amount: **10.00**
Co-Pay Note: Leave blank

Click **Submit**.

Entity/Payers: Select

Note at top of screen: "Payer attached to patient..."

Click **Exit Screen**.

Patient/Payers

Place cursor in box next to "South Padre Insurance Company."
Click **Confirm Payers**.

Visit Add screen

Type of Visit: **Doctor**

Payment Information

Amount: **10.00 (Note: must include .00)**
Type: **Cash**
Source: **Patient**
Note: Leave blank

Click **Submit**.

Visit Add screen

Reason for Visit: States **"Sprained right ankle"**
Type of Visit: Click down arrow and select **Doctor**.

Click Submit.

Nursing Note Add screen

Click **Injury-Muscles**.
Click **Submit**.

Screen to select the body part or parts injured

Select the right ankle.
Hit **ENTER** on keyboard.
Click **Exit Screen** to return the Patients screen.
Go to Main Menu.
Click **Clinic Status**.

You will see that Mark Bogert is now waiting for physician. The screen returns to the patient database, where you confirm by hitting **ENTER** on your keyboard. The patient is now successfully registered.

Next walk-in patient:

SSN:	**204-59-6432**
Patient:	**Don Burthold**
Address:	**1816 Gulfstream Drive**
	South Padre, TX 98765
Telephone:	**209-555-0809**
DOB:	**10/22/1971**
Gender:	**Male**
Marital Status:	**Married**

Click **Submit**.
Press **ENTER** if correct or **F3** to change.

Companies

Click **Patient Responsibility**.
Select **Company**.

New Case

Complaint:	**Left shoulder pain**

Click **Submit**.

Entity/Payers: Select

Insurance:	**Texas Health Corporation**

Click **Select Payer**.

Patient/Payer

Subscriber Relationship:	**Self**
Last Name:	**Burthold**
First Name:	**Don**
Middle Initial:	Leave blank
DOB:	**10/22/1971**
Gender:	**Male**
Policy Effective:	**10/06/08**
Termination:	Leave blank
ID #:	**MYT8822**
Group Name:	**ELSTX**
Group #:	**P2900**
Plan Type:	**Basic**
Co-Insurance %:	**20%**
Co-Pay Amount:	**20.00**
Co-Pay Note:	Leave blank

Click **Submit**.

DAY EIGHT TASK 8.1

Entity/Payers: Select

Note at top of screen: "Payer attached to patient..."
Click **Exit Screen**.

Patient/Payers

Place cursor in command box next to "South Padre Insurance Company."
Click **Confirm Payers**.

Visit Add

Type of Visit: **Doctor**

Payment Information

Amount: **20.00**
Type: **Cash**
Source: **Patient**

Click **Submit**.

Nursing Note Add screen

Click **Injury-Muscles**.
Click **Submit**.

Screen to select the body part or parts

Select the left shoulder.
Hit **ENTER** on keyboard.
Click **Exit Screen** to return to the Patients screen.
Go to Main Menu.
Click **Clinic Status**.

You will see that Don Burthold is now waiting for physician. The screen returns to the patient database, where you confirm by hitting **ENTER** on your keyboard. The patient is now successfully registered.

Next walk-in patient:

SSN:	**207-77-9843**
Patient:	**Dan Dore**
Address:	**6000 Willow Way**
	South Padre, TX 98765
Telephone:	**209-555-6714**
DOB:	**12/24/1953**
Gender:	**Male**
Marital Status:	**Married**

Click **Submit**.
Press **ENTER** if correct or **F3** to change.

Companies

Click **Patient Responsibility**.
Select **Company**.

New Case

Complaint:	**Lower back pain**

Click **Submit**.

Entity/Payers: Select

Insurance:	**BC/BS of Texas**

Click **Select Payer**.

Patient/Payer

Subscriber Relationship:	**Self**
Last name:	**Dore**
First name:	**Dan**
DOB:	**12/24/1953**
Gender:	**M**
Policy Effective:	**05/06/07**
ID #:	**CXZ4848**
Group Name:	**Basic**
Group #:	**Z4812**
Plan Type:	**Basic**
Co-Insurance %:	**20%**
Co-Pay Amount:	**25.00**

Click **Submit**.

DAY EIGHT TASK 8.1

Entity/Payers: Select

Note at top of screen: "Payer attached to patient…"

Click **Exit Screen**.

Patient/Payers

Place cursor in command box next to "South Padre Insurance Company."
Click **Confirm Payers**.

Visit Add

Type of Visit: **Doctor**

Payment Information

Amount: **25.00**
Type: **Cash**
Source: **Patient**

Click **Submit**.

Nursing Note Add

Click **Injury-Muscles**.
Click **Submit**.

Screen to select the lower back

Hit **ENTER** on keyboard.
Click **Exit Screen**.
Go to Main Menu.
Click **Clinic Status**.

You will see that Dan Dore is now a patient in the waiting room. The screen returns to the patient database, where you confirm by hitting **ENTER** on your keyboard. The patient is now successfully registered.

Task **8.2**

ACCESSING AND PRINTING ONLINE CHARTS

From the Main Menu, click **Patient Registration** to access the patient database. Next, place your cursor in the field next to Dianne G. Barron's name, key in "date," and press **ENTER**. The display that you will see shows the date that Dianne was placed into the MedTrak system. Place your cursor in the command box next to her name and click the **On-line Chart** link on the left side of the screen. This is the EHR for Dianne, which you created when you registered her. The nursing staff will add to this information as they complete the intake work on the patient (e.g., blood pressure, height, and weight). The physician will then add to the EHR with additional information. There is a Function command box above the Diagnoses in Dianne's online chart. In the Function box type "prch" and press **ENTER** on your keyboard. This command sends a copy of the patient online chart to the View Prints section of the system. Click the **Exit Chart** link on the left side of the screen. This takes you back one screen, which has a View Prints link on the left. Click that link, locate the chart you just printed, and save a copy to your Completed Work folder as LastName_YourFirstInitial_Task8.2Barron.

Exit back to the Main Menu. Gladys wants you to save a copy of the online chart of the other patients you registered in the MedTrak system. She asks you to use the **Clinic Status** screen to access the patient record by clicking Clinic Status on the main screen. Then place your cursor next to the patient whose chart you want to print and click the **Online Chart** button on the left side of the screen. Gladys wants you to see that there are several ways to access the chart. Save the charts into the Completed Work folder as follows:

Mark Bogert: LastName_YourFirstInitial_Task8.2Bogert

Don Burthold: LastName_YourFirstInitial_Task8.2Burthold

Dan Dore: LastName_YourFirstInitial_Task8.2Dore

Now Gladys wants you to print the online chart for Liz Furry. Access the chart from the Main Menu, Patient Registration, and locate Liz's entry in the database. Then, in succession, click **Select Patient, Show Cases, Visit Log,** and **Online Chart**. Type "PRCH" (case does not matter) in the Function box and press **ENTER**. Click **Exit Chart** and then click **View Prints** to see, open, and save a copy of the online chart. Save a copy of Liz's chart to your Completed Work folder as LastName_YourFirstInitial_Task8.2Furry.

Using the directions for printing Liz's online chart, print and save the online charts for the following:

- Dianna Morris (DOS: 04/16/12)—save as LastName_YourFirstInitial_Task8.2Morris
- Kenny Gilbertson (DOS: 03/05/12)—save as LastName_YourFirstInitial_Task8.2Gilbertson
- Brenda Threewings (DOS: 04/16/12)—save as LastName_YourFirstInitial_Task8.2Threewings
- Kim Zahn (DOS: 04/16/12)—save as LastName_YourFirstInitial_Task8.2Zahn
- Arty Giddings (DOS: 04/16/12)—save as LastName_YourFirstInitial_Task8.2Giddings
- Li Wong (DOS: 04/17/12)—save as LastName_YourFirstInitial_Task8.2Wong

Exercise 8-1

Using the online charts you just saved to your Completed Work folder, answer the following questions:

1. The Orders section of Liz Furry's chart indicates this dosage of toradol: _____.

2. Dianne Morris' father died at the age of _____.

3. Kenny Gilbertson is _____ years old.

4. Brenda Threewings' weight is _____ pounds.

5. Kim Zahn received _____ mg of Soma during her 04/16/12 office visit.

Task **8.3**

RECORDING AND TOTALING DAILY RECEIPTS

You are now going to print the Patient Payment Log. From the Main Menu, click the **Reports Menu** tab. This tab displays the various reports that the Center uses to track activities. For example, as you have been at the front desk receiving money from patients, you entered those payments in the MedTrak system. At the end of your time at the front desk, you must account for the funds you received. The system has been keeping track of what you have been entering as payments from each patient. From the Reports Menu, click **Print Patient Payment Log,** and when the next screen displays, you can either accept the date shown or enter another date, accept the default (today's date) and click **Print** at the bottom of the dialog box. When you do this, red text reading "Report sent to printer..." appears above the box. Exit the screen to return to the Reports Menu, where you click the **View Prints** button on the left side of the screen. Open the payment summary document and save a copy to your Completed Work folder as LastName_YourFirstInitial_Task8.3Payments. In the office, print a copy of this log and balance the coins, cash, checks, and credit card receipts that you took in against the log. Then enter the grand total and sign your name. Another staff member must verify the total against the log and sign the form on the "Verified by" line on the log. This log is then used in the preparation of the daily deposits, which are done by Kerri Marshall. After you have signed the form, Gladys will verify the form and the funds will be given to Kerri for deposit. You must be very careful with the money, checks, and credit card receipts you receive because you will be accountable to balance these against the log.

Task **8.4**

ACCESSING NPIs AND SSNs

As your last task of the day with Gladys, you will learn more about the MedTrak system. From the Main Menu, click the **User Menu** tab on the right of the screen. Click **Consultants**, the first button on the User Menu screen. Displayed are all of the consultants to whom the physicians refer patients. Click the green **Page Down** arrow and then click the green **Page Up** arrow to return to the top of the list. Links along the left side of the screen allow you to add, change, delete, and "un-delete" consultants. You can also sort the list by name, city, zip code, or type order. Place your cursor in the command box next to "John Andrews" and click the **More Functions** link on the left side of the screen. Here you will see not only the Command Help functions that appeared as links on the previous screen (such as Add and Change), but also other functions that were not available as links (such as ID Numbers). Click the box next to "ID Numbers" and click **Select Function** on the left side of the screen. A screen will appear on which you change the NPI (National Physician Identification) number. Dr. Andrews' number is 2139464141. Exit the screen displaying Dr. Andrews' NPI number.

Exercise 8-2

Display the consultants' NPI numbers to answer these questions:

1. Dr. McDonald's NPI number is _____.

2. Dr. Bethos' NPI number is _____.

3. Dr. Blackburn's NPI number is _____.

From the Main Menu, click the **Search Menu** tab to display the various searches you can do within the system. You can search by case, companies, visits by date, patients, or SSN. Let's do some searches by SSN. Click the **SSN** button to display the patient in numeric order by SSN. Using the SSN search feature, answer the questions in the following exercise.

Exercise 8-3

Match the patient name to the correct SSN.

1. 201-48-9201	a. Gus Conrad
2. 405-45-5404	b. Jackie L. King
3. 448-61-8102	c. Amanda J. Foster
4. 502-44-8754	d. Lewis L. Rock
5. 311-64-7841	e. Fran Jacques

Yet another day in your internship is finished! Time is moving quickly—you only have two days left and the last day is devoted to closing out your internship. Gladys has tasks left for you to do, but you have learned so much today that she will allow you to check out. Don't forget to keep your Equipment Maintenance and Desk Security form current, because you will have to hand that form in to your supervisor at the end of your internship.

You have just one final task before you are finished for this day—take the following short ten-question quiz.

Quiz

DAY 8

Using the MedTrak software, answer the following questions:

1. Dianne Barron presented with what complaint?
   a. Back pain
   b. Wrist strain
   c. Headache
   d. Ankle sprain

2. Mark Bogert presented with what complaint?
   a. Back pain
   b. Wrist strain
   c. Headache
   d. Ankle sprain

3. According to Liz Furry's medical record, Dr. Adams' Impression section of the 04/16/12 report indicated acute sinusitis and which of the following?
   a. Headache
   b. Flu
   c. Bronchitis
   d. Depression

4. The diagnosis code reported for Brenda Threewings 04/16/12 office visit was which of the following?
   a. 300.00
   b. 307.81
   c. V17.1
   d. 465.9

5. Using the Search feature, to which patient does the SSN 506-80-8000 belong?
   a. Jasper Hunt
   b. Amanda Foster
   c. Anthony Anglea
   d. Alice Cummings

6. According to Arty Giddings' online chart, for the 04/16/12 office visit, her past, family, and social history indicates hypothyroidism and what other condition?
   a. Diabetes
   b. Chronic headaches
   c. Mental illness
   d. Tubal ligation

7. According to Li Wong's online chart, what is her age?
   a. 55
   b. 61
   c. 32
   d. 46

8. According to the Patient Payment Log you printed, what was the grand total of funds received for 04/18/12?
   a. $62
   b. $55
   c. $20
   d. $85

9. When you access the User Menu and search the database of consultants, what is Dr. Bethos' NPI number?
   a. 3120981143
   b. 3120981155
   c. 3120981144
   d. 3120981644

10. Who is the person responsible for making the Center's daily bank deposits and who ultimately receives the Patient Payment Log?
    a. You
    b. Kerri Marshall
    c. Gladys Johnson
    d. Jennifer White

It's time to receive credit for your quiz! Remember that you **must** go to the Scheduler, type "**QUIZ**" in any command line, and press **ENTER**. The next screen you will see displays a box that says "I am done with the Quiz for Day 8." If you are done, click **Yes**. If you have not completed the quiz, click **No** and you will be returned to the Scheduler. After you have clicked the **Yes** button on the Day 8 Quiz dialog box, your screen will display **Day 8 completed, Day 9 (April 19, 2012) charts loaded**.

DAY EIGHT QUIZ

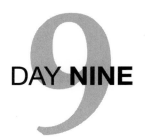

DAY NINE

Thursday, April 19, 2012

TASK **9.1**	Uploading EHR Documents
TASK **9.2**	Scheduling Call-Ins
TASK **9.3**	Processing Accounts Receivable

TASK **9.1**

UPLOADING EHR DOCUMENTS

 Supplies Located on Evolve

- 14 medical documents

Gladys wants you to begin the day by uploading the documents for surgical patients from yesterday, Wednesday, April 18. She knows you have performed this tasks many times in the past (remember "doc"), so she only tells you the order in which she wants the documents uploaded:

- Anthony Anglea, Emergency Department
- Anthony Anglea, Hospital Admit
- Anthony Anglea, Radiology Report
- Anthony Anglea, Cardiac Catheterization
- Anthony Anglea, Angioplasty/Stenting
- Lonnie Carson, Operative Report
- Emily Fisk, Operative Report
- William Foley, Operative Report
- Mike Gillian, Operative Report
- Dave Kuhn, Operative Report
- Robin Kupeck, Cardiac Catheterization
- Robin Kupeck, Radiology Report
- Robin Kupeck, Angioplasty/Stent
- Ti Wong, Echocardiogram

Task **9.2**

SCHEDULING CALL-INS

- Silvia Scott calls in early in the morning and wants to be scheduled for an appointment with Dr. Adams. She recently established Dr. Adams as a primary care physician and now has an ingrown toenail that kept her awake last night. She wants to come in as soon as she can. Schedule her for the first open appointment on Dr. Adams' schedule for today.

- Adam Hoverson calls in right after Silvia and also wants to see Dr. Adams today as early as possible. He was in to see Dr. Adams on 04/09/12 for problems with his ears, and he says the doctor told him that if he didn't get better in two weeks, he should come in again. There has been no change in Mr. Hoverson's condition, so he wants to see Dr. Adams because his ear infection is not better.

- It's a busy morning! Right after you hang up the telephone, it rings again. This time, Anne Meires is calling; she wants to see Dr. Adams as soon as she can. She says her dizziness is not better and she really wants to get in to see the doctor today as early as you can get her in.

- The next call is from David Oakland, who is having neck pain and wants to see Dr. Adams as soon as possible because the pain is so severe that he has not been able to go to work today.

- Sylvia Kennedy calls and wants to have her ears washed out today. She wants to see Dr. Adams if possible.

Gladys wants you to save a copy of Dr. Adams schedule for today in your Completed Work folder as LastName_YourFirstInitial_Task9.2Adams.

Task 9.3

PROCESSING ACCOUNTS RECEIVABLE

It is time to process the accounts receivable. Recall that from the Main Menu, you access the accounts by clicking the **Billing** button and then the **Unbilled Dashboard** button. Gladys has reviewed the "Completed Visits, Charges available for review, Patient" and wants you to post all the charges for her. When you are finished, there should be no charges in the Completed Visits charges area because you will have posted all the charges.

Next, Gladys asks you to access the "Bills ready to be Processed" screen using the Billing Menu. Now that you have posted all the charges, there are 14 insurance patients to bill and 7 patient invoices to prepare. View and print the bills for the 14 CMS-1500 patients. With the "Invoices, Unprinted, CMS-1500's, Not Bill Elec" displayed on your screen, click the down arrow next to "Change Payer Display" and select **All Payers** from the drop-down menu. Next, click the down arrow to the left of "Change Display Order" and select **Patient** to view the patients as listed in Figure 9-1.

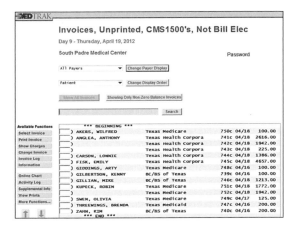

Figure 9-1: Invoices sorted alphabetically by patient

The first patient is Wilfred Akers, who was seen on 04/18/12 and has $100 in charges to send to his insurance company, Texas Medicare. Select his invoice by placing your cursor in the command box next to his name and clicking the **Print Invoice** button on the left side of your screen. Save a copy of Wilfred Akers' CMS-1500 in your Completed Work folder as LastName_YourFirstInitial_Task9.3Akers.

Print the invoices on the remaining patients and save as follows:

- LastName_YourFirstInitial_Task9.3Anglea1
- LastName_YourFirstInitial_Task9.3Anglea2
- LastName_YourFirstInitial_Task9.3Anglea3
- LastName_YourFirstInitial_Task9.3Carson
- LastName_YourFirstInitial_Task9.3Fisk
- LastName_YourFirstInitial_Task9.3Giddings
- LastName_YourFirstInitial_Task9.3Gilbertson
- LastName_YourFirstInitial_Task9.3Gillian
- LastName_YourFirstInitial_Task9.3Kupeck1
- LastName_YourFirstInitial_Task9.3Kupeck2
- LastName_YourFirstInitial_Task9.3Swen
- LastName_YourFirstInitial_Task9.3Threewings
- LastName_YourFirstInitial_Task9.3Zahn

After you have saved each of the CMS-1500s for the above patients, exit back to the "Bills ready to be Processed" screen. You will see that there are 0s in the "Insurance - CMS-1500" area because you have successfully processed the forms.

Move on to the seven patient invoices that you are to print. Save a copy of each invoice in your Completed Work folder as follows:

- LastName_YourFirstInitial_Task9.3Furry
- LastName_YourFirstInitial_Task9.3Kolpeck
- LastName_YourFirstInitial_Task9.3Morris
- LastName_YourFirstInitial_Task9.3Nuson
- LastName_YourFirstInitial_Task9.3Schultz
- LastName_YourFirstInitial_Task9.3Li Wong
- LastName_YourFirstInitial_Task9.3Ti Wong

When you exit back to the "Bills ready to be Processed" screen, you will see that there are no patients in the "Patient - Invoices" area to be processed. You have successfully processed all the bills and the insurance forms and printed the invoices. Good job!

Exercise 9-1

Using the documents you saved from the tasks you have completed in Day 9, answer the following questions.

1. Anne Meires' insurance company is _____.

2. The charge for Wilfred Akers' 04/18/12 office visit was _____.

3. Lillian Schultz's invoice indicates that her street address is _____.

4. Is the address for Ti Wong and Li Wong the same? _____

You have just one final task before you are finished for this day—take the following short ten-question quiz.

Quiz

DAY 9

Using the MedTrak software, answer the following questions:

1. David Oakland was scheduled with Dr. Adams on 04/19/12 for what complaint?
   a. Ingrown toenail
   b. Ear infection
   c. Dizziness
   d. Neck pain

2. Anne Meires was scheduled with Dr. Adams on 04/19/12 for what complaint?
   a. Ingrown toenail
   b. Ear infection
   c. Dizziness
   d. Neck pain

3. Wilfred Akers' insurance company is which of the following?
   a. Texas Medicare
   b. Texas Health Corporation
   c. BC/BS of Texas
   d. Texas Medicaid

4. Brenda Threewings' insurance company is which of the following?
   a. Texas Medicare
   b. Texas Health Corporation
   c. BC/BS of Texas
   d. Texas Medicaid

5. What is the amount of Mrs. Li Wong's invoice?
   a. $224
   b. $110
   c. $120
   d. $130

6. What is the amount of Liz Furry's invoice?
   a. $224
   b. $110
   c. $120
   d. $130

7. Dr. Adams' 04/19/12 schedule indicates he is _____ from 1-3 p.m.
   a. Conducting rounds
   b. Seeing office patients
   c. At the medical school
   d. Unavailable

8. According to the operative report you uploaded to Lonnie Carson's EHR, on 04/18/12, Dr. Bond performed which procedure?
   a. Appendectomy
   b. Right knee replacement
   c. Menisectomy
   d. Cholecystectomy

DAY NINE QUIZ

9. According to the operative report you uploaded into Mike Gillian's EHR, on 04/18/12, Dr. Clark performed which procedure?
    a. Appendectomy
    b. Right knee replacement
    c. Menisectomy
    d. Cholecystectomy

10. The CPT code listed on Kenny Gilbertson's CMS-1500 is which of the following?
    a. 99210
    b. 99213
    c. 99202
    d. 99214

It's time to receive credit for your quiz! Remember that you **must** go to the Scheduler, type "**QUIZ**" in any command line, and press **ENTER**. The next screen you will see displays a box that says "I am done with the Quiz for Day 9." If you are done, click **Yes**. If you have not completed the quiz, click **No** and you will be returned to the Scheduler. After you have clicked the **Yes** button on the Day 9 Quiz dialog box, your screen will display **Day 9 completed, Day 10 (April 20, 2012) charts loaded**.

10 DAY TEN

Friday, April 20, 2012

TASK **10.1**	Uploading Documents
TASK **10.2**	Scheduling Appointments
TASK **10.3**	Updating Consultant NPIs
TASK **10.4**	Wrap-Up

TASK **10.1**

UPLOADING DOCUMENTS

Supplies Located on Evolve

- 2 medical documents

Well here it is, the last day of your internship! Didn't the time go fast? Gladys shares with you that she thinks this time has gone quickly and she can hardly believe it is already Day 10 and your last internship day. There are still a few things Gladys wants you to learn and do before you are finished for the day, but she knows those first few days were especially long, so this day will be especially short to make up for that!

Download two operative reports from the Evolve website—one for Jason Eskew and one for Edward Goldman. Upload these documents to the patient's EHR.

Task **10.2**

SCHEDULING APPOINTMENTS

Max Foster is a walk-in patient, and Gladys asks you to register him with Dr. Adams at 9 a.m. today. Mr. Foster's complaint is a suspected sexually transmitted disease (STD).

SSN:	**274-66-9087**
Name:	**Mr. Max Foster**
Address:	**1603 Todd Avenue**
	South Padre, TX 98765
Home Telephone:	**209-555-7767**
DOB:	**07/18/1991**
Gender:	**Male**
Marital Status:	**Married**
Type of Visit:	**Doctor**
Insurance:	**South Padre Insurance Company**
	2702 Oak Line Drive
	South Padre, TX 98765
Relationship:	**Self**
Effective:	**01/01/90**
Term Date:	Leave blank
ID #:	**PJD9123**
Group Name:	**PPS**
Group #:	**40005**
Plan Type:	**PPS**
Co-Insurance %:	**20%**
Co-Pay Amount:	**25**
Payment:	**Cash**

Make a copy of the patient chart you just created for Max Foster and save a copy to your Completed Work folder as LastName_YourFirstInitial_Task10.2Foster.

The next walk-in patient is also for Dr. Adams. This patient is Emmy L. Harkland, who presents with hip pain and wants to be seen as soon as possible. She fell down at home early this morning and has had pain in the right hip since that time.

SSN:	**009-99-0099**
Name:	**Mrs. Emmy L. Harkland**
Address:	**1818 Oak Street**
	South Padre, TX 98765
Home Telephone:	**209-555-5209**
DOB:	**04/06/1946**
Gender:	**Female**
Marital Status:	**Widow**
Type of Visit:	**Doctor**
Insurance:	**Texas Medicare**
	402 Main Street
	South Padre, TX 98765
Relationship:	**Self**
Effective:	**04/06/01**
Term Date:	Leave blank
ID #	009990099A
Group Name:	**Medicare**
Group #:	009990099A
Plan Type:	**Part A**
Co-Insurance %:	**20%**
Co-Pay Amount:	**20**
Payment:	**Cash**

Make a copy of the patient chart you just created for Emmy Harkland and save a copy to your Completed Work folder as LastName_YourFirstInitial_Task10.2Harkland.

Task **10.3**

UPDATING CONSULTANT NPIs

NPIs (National Provider Identification) are 10-digit numbers that are issued on a national level and are unique to each provider. Gladys asks you to verify the consultant NPI numbers for her. Recall that you access the list of consultants from the User Menu by clicking on the **Consultants** button. Next to the first physician on the list of consultants is John Andrews. Place your cursor in the command box next to his name, key in "ID" and press **ENTER** on your keyboard. When you do this, Dr. Andrews' name appears in green at the top of the screen, and his NPI number appears below that. Click the **Exit Screen** link on the left side to return to the list of consultants. The following are the names and NPI numbers that Gladys wants you to look up; verify that the NPI numbers are correctly listed for each physician.

	Type	**ID Number**
Louis Argabright	NPI	7658421001
Gregory Dawson	NPI	9284501192
Robert Evans	NPI	1234098532
Larry P. Friendly	NPI	5945782309
Ethan Green	NPI	3232490845
Harry Greggory	NPI	3498102384

When you are finished verifying the NPI numbers with the physician names, Gladys wants you to print a copy of the consultants. From the User Menu, click the **Consultants** button to display the list of consultants. Click the **More Functions** button, the **Print** check box, and the **Select Function** link on the left. A dialog box will open, requesting you to input the alphabetic range. Type "a" in the "Beg" block and "z" in the "End" block; then click **Print** on the dialog box. The report will go to the View Prints area, so exit the screen until you have returned to a screen where the View Prints link is displayed. Click **View Prints** and locate the consultant list you just printed. Save a copy to your Completed Work folder as LastName_YourFirstInitial_Task10.3Consult.

Task **10.4**

WRAP-UP

Well, it is the end of your internship. We, at the Center, all wish you the very best of luck in your career. We think that you are an excellent intern and have accomplished a great deal in your two weeks with us. We hope that you have enjoyed your time with us and that you keep us in mind when you are choosing your future employer. You have been an asset to the Center. Don't forget to return your keys to Gladys before you leave and make certain you have retrieved your personal belongs from the locker and desk. Gladys wants you to print a copy of your Equipment and Desk Security form and leave it with her on your way out. Again, we hope you have enjoyed your time at the Center.

Before you leave, your only task left is to take the following short ten-question quiz.

Quiz

DAY 10

Using the MedTrak software, answer the following questions:

1. What is Wilfred Akers' date of birth?
   a. 05/22/1952
   b. 06/13/1940
   c. 01/28/2008
   d. 04/23/1935

2. Fred Bass' street address is which of the following?
   a. 501 Clam
   b. 590 West Ward
   c. 9340 Mission Street
   d. 5252 Westward Drive

3. Alice Cummings' SSN is which of the following?
   a. 506-80-8000
   b. 204-58-3621
   c. 501-68-1786
   d. 001-13-4982

4. Dr. Theodore Blackburn's NPI number is which of the following?
   a. 9870238510
   b. 6578184377
   c. 7792554111
   d. 7739745986

5. According to the schedule for 04/20/12, Dr. Harkness' schedule is matrixed as which of the following?
   a. Surgery
   b. Unavailable
   c. Medical school
   d. Office patients

6. From the Main Menu, which button would you click first if you wanted to review Unbilled Charges?
   a. Clinic Status
   b. Patient Registration
   c. Billing
   d. User Menu

7. From the Main Menu, which button would you click first if you wanted to upload a document to a patient's EHR by keying "doc" next to their name?
   a. Clinic Status
   b. Patient Registration
   c. Billing
   d. User Menu

8. When you view the documents that have been attached to Floyd Barr's EHR, what document do you not see in the list of attached documents?
   a. Angioplasty/Stenting
   b. Cardiac Catheterization
   c. Operative Report
   d. Admission

9. When you view the documents attached to Anthony Anglea's EHR, one of them is an "Admission" that was done by Dr. Harkness on which date?
   a. 04/17/12
   b. 04/12/12
   c. 04/18/12
   d. 04/09/12

10. From the Main Menu, which tab would you click first in order to make a referral?
    a. Pending Menu
    b. Reports Menu
    c. Search Menu
    d. User Menu

Time to receive credit for your quiz. Remember that you **must** go to the Scheduler, type "**QUIZ**" in any command line, and press **ENTER** on your keyboard. The screen will display "no more quizzes." This means you are finished! CONGRATULATIONS!

Appendix A—Appointment Scheduling Guidelines

15 MINUTES
- Allergies
- Bug bite
- Burn
- Cast recheck
- Conjunctivitis
- Cough
- Ear pain or infection
- Ear wash
- Elevated temperature
- Fall recheck
- Flu symptoms
- Pharyngitis
- Rash, hives
- Recheck flu
- Recheck Pap
- Sinus
- Sore throat
- URI
- UTI
- Wart treatment

30 MINUTES
- Abdominal pain
- Asthma
- Anxiety
- Back pain recheck
- Breast mass
- Bronchitis
- Cast change
- Chest congestion
- Chest pain
- Confusion
- Depression
- Diabetic new problem
- Diabetic recheck
- Dizziness
- Eye injury
- Foreign body removal (location)
- Headache
- Hernia
- Hip pain recheck
- Infection
- Ingrown toenail
- Laceration, head, arm, hand
- Leg pain recheck
- Lesion removal (1)
- Medication recheck
- Menstrual problems

- Muscle strain
- OB check
- Pap
- Postoperative visit
- Preop physical
- Shortness of breath (SOB)
- Sprain or suspected fracture
- STD
- Stiff neck
- Varicocele recheck

45 MINUTES
- Back pain
- Breast pain
- Dog bite
- Hip pain
- Knee pain
- Laceration, trunk, leg
- Leg pain
- Lump
- Neck pain
- Shoulder pain
- Varicose veins
- Postoperative complication or pain

60 MINUTES
- Establish physician
- Initial OB

PHYSICALS/PAPS
15 to 60 MINUTES
- Pap included for female patients (over age 18)
- Physicals (px) and preoperatives (preop) (schedule by age)

Under 18	15 minutes
18-40	30 minutes
41-65	45 minutes
Over 65	60 minutes

CONSULTATION
Request for an inpatient consultation: Prefer an hour but can schedule for 45 minutes. Note reason for consultation and requesting physician when placing inpatient consultation on schedule.

CARDIAC 1 HOUR
- New cardiac outpatient
- New inpatient consultation

SURGERY SCHEDULING
45 MINUTES
- Cholecystectomy, laparoscopic
- Fracture repair
- Hearing check
- Lesion removal (2 or more)
- Outpatient echocardiogram
- Proctosigmoidoscopy (procto)
- Hernia repair

60 MINUTES
- Appendectomy, laparoscopic
- Breast biopsy
- Cardiac catheterization
- Hernia repair with graft
- Initial (new) OB visit
- Kidney biopsy
- Liver biopsy
- Lymph biopsy
- Lymphadenectomy
- Mastectomy
- Needle biopsy
- New surgical patient
- Pacemaker
- Septoplasty
- Surgical echocardiogram

90 MINUTES
- Decompression, arthroscopic, such as, shoulder
- Discectomy
- GI bypass, laparoscopic
- Microdiscectomy

120 MINUTES
- Hip, closed reduction and screw placement
- Knee, total arthroplasty
- Meniscectomy
- Laminectomy, foraminotomies, facetectomies
- Tendon, open repair

Appendix B—Business Directory

Information

John Andrews, MD

Louis Argabright, MD

Bert Bethos, MD
  209-555-8231

Theodore Blackburn, MD

Robert Evans, MD

Ethan Green, MD

Harry Greggory, MD

Clarence McDonald, MD
  209-555-8292

Stafford Morgan, MD

Rush Peters, MD

Dennis Smith, MD Fort Worth

Morton Samson, MD
  1256 56th Avenue South
  Houston TX 99881
  956-934-6120

Thomas Thompson, MD
  209-555-0090

Business Information

First National Bank
South Padre TX 98765
100 First Street

South Padre Medical Center
9878 Palm Drive
South Padre TX 98765
209-555-3356

South Padre Hospital
980 Lagona Drive
South Padre TX 98765
209-555-4289

South Padre Surgery Center
209-555-8247

Texas Health Corporation
1256 56th Avenue South
Houston TX 99881

Texas Health Corporation
884 Worthington Rd
San Antonio TX 99784

Appendix C—Exercise Answers

Exercise P-1:
1. c
2. b

Exercise P-2:
1. m
2. m
3. d
4. a
5. f
6. f
7. i
8. e
9. b
10. k
11. c
12. j
13. g
14. l
15. h

Exercise P-3:
1. Jeffrey, Edna
2. 209-555-9224

Exercise P-4:
1. Blair, Thomas R.
2. Rock, Lewis
3. Ramona

Exercise 2-1:
1. 04/18/12, 3:00p
2. 04/10/12, 1:00p, Bond
3. 04/10/12, 2:30p, Adams
4. 04/11/12, 10:15a, Adams

Exercise 2-2:
1. BLT6446
2. back and leg pn
3. 2:15p
4. breast mass

Exercise 3-1:
1. left
2. 02/14/10
3. left hip
4. 200

Exercise 3-2:
1. insurance
2. Dr. Clark
3. Dr. Bond
4. accounts receivable

Exercise 4-1:
1. Smith, Carol
   04/09/12 **11:30a** Bond, Gerald
   04/12/12 3:00p Bond, Gerald
2. Terry Emily Greggory
   04/09/12 12:15p Bond, Gerald
   04/**12**/12 1:00p Bond, Gerald
3. William J. Foley
   04/09/12 1:00p **Adams, Ray**
   04/18/12 9:00a Clark, Anthony
4. Jackie W. Masci
   04/09/12 **4:15p** Adams, Ray
   04/12/12 2:45p Clark, Anthony
5. Edward **A.** Goldman
   04/10/12 2:30p Bond, Gerald
   04/19/12 1:00p Bond, Gerald
6. Eugena Dore
   04/10/12 8:00a Adams, Ray
   04/10/12 8:00a Bond, Gerald
   04/10/12 **3:45p** **Bond, Gerald**
7. Jasper Hunt
   04/10/**12** 2:30p Adams, Ray
   04/19/**12** 10:00a Adams, Ray
8. Lori H. Whittaker
   04/11/12 8:00a **Bond, Gerald**
   04/11/12 2:00p Bond, Gerald
9. Andy Andrews
   04/11/12 10:30a Bond, Gerald
   04/20/12 1:00p Bond, Gerald
10. Jason W. Eskew
    04/11/12 11:15a Bond, Gerald
    04/19/12 3:0**0p** Bond, Gerald
11. Eloise Fisher
    04/**09**/12 11:00a Bond, Gerald
    04/11/12 1:00p Bond, Gerald
12. Harriet Muir
    04/11/12 **4:00p** Harkness, Joyce
    04/12/12 12:00p Harkness, Joyce
13. Floyd Barr
    0**4**/11/12 8:00a Harkness, Joyce
    04/11/12 11:00a Harkness, Joyce

Exercise 4-2:
1. closed
2. unstable
3. general
4. Bert Bethos, MD

Exercise 6-1:

1. **Hello, Mr. Johnson?** (Always get a confirmation of whom you are speaking to—never leave information with anyone other than the patient.) **This is "Your Name" from the South Padre Medical Center. I am returning your call regarding an appointment with Dr. Bond for Wednesday, April 18. We have reserved an appointment for you on Wednesday, April 18, at 9 a.m. Is this time convenient for you?** (assuming the patient said it was a convenient time) **Our offices are located at 9878 Palm Drive in South Padre.** (Always ask if they know how to locate the office.) **Please bring along any medications you are currently taking and your insurance card(s). We look forward to seeing you on Wednesday, April 18, at 9 a.m. If you have any questions in the meantime, call us at 555-4298.**

Exercise 7-1:

1. $50
2. 09/15
3. Visa
4. septoplasty

Exercise 7-2:

1. $6,166
2. $1,899
3. 7
4. 3

Exercise 8-1:

1. 60 mg
2. 62
3. 45
4. 171
5. 350

Exercise 8-2:

1. 5925442862
2. 3120981144
3. 7739745986

Exercise 8-3:

1. d
2. e
3. b
4. c
5. a

Exercise 9-1:

1. Texas Health Corporation
2. $100
3. 17 Hillside
4. yes